T0270518

Praise for *Unavoidably Unsafe*

"Driven by long standing vaccine ideology, hubris, and profits, the routine childhood vaccine schedule has grown exponentially in the absence of new and substantial infectious disease threats to children. Mounting evidence over decades suggests the theoretical benefits of vaccines may have been outweighed by real harms rendering the entire program 'unavoidably unsafe.' Drs. Geehr and Barke help parents navigate this new reality, going shot by shot, providing the information needed for full informed consent. This guide is destined to be a valuable resource for every young family and a wonderful companion for pediatric well-baby visits."

—Peter A. McCullough, MD, MPH, Internal Medicine, Cardiology, Dallas TX, and author of *Courage to Face COVID-19: Preventing Hospitalization and Death While Battling the Bio-Pharmaceutical Complex*

"Drs. Edward Geehr and Jeffrey Barke present an incredibly well-written treatise documenting irrefutable evidence of the absolute corruption of the fraudulent governmental-pharmaceutical vaccine complex. This is a must read for all global citizens including every physician. This masterpiece not only presents data that cannot be discounted, but also a fascinating history of the vaccines. The brainwashing, mind control, and corporate kleptocracy has been completed through every stitch of the tapestry of our society. We were taught nothing in medical school about vaccines except to always give them and that they were proven safe and effective. Jonas Salk visited our medical school class, and he was revered as a god. Drs. Geehr and Barke expose the typical revolving door between the pharmaceutical industry and the federal regulators exactly as depicted so recently with Scott Gottlieb serving as the 23rd Commissioner of the FDA and now with Pfizer. This book is riveting!"

—James A .Thorp, MD, board certified in Ob/Gyn and in sub-specialty maternal-fetal medicine, Chief of Maternal and Prenatal Health, The Wellness Company at TWC@health

"Vaccination status has become nearly as divisive a topic as religion and politics. This excellent new book couldn't have come at a better time! With authority and clarity, the authors dispel vaccine myths, expose the Judas character of many in the pharmaceutical industry, and show us all how to get the power of our families' health back into the hands of 'we the people.' If you want to understand the true story behind vaccines, their value, and their risks, give this book a shot."

—Kirk Cameron, actor, producer, and evangelist

"*Unavoidably Unsafe* is co-authored by two physicians who have dedicated over three decades to the practice of medicine and encapsulates not just the breadth of their medical knowledge, but also the depth of their commitment to truth. While we currently witness the wide-scale intersection of medicine and policy, Dr. Barke and Dr. Geehr's insights into childhood vaccines show their unwavering dedication to the principles of individual freedom and informed healthcare decisions. Their book is more than a collection of facts from a seasoned physician; it is a call to action for any parent who is considering vaccines for their children. It challenges parents to think critically and do research before allowing their children to be injected with a product that could potentially be detrimental to their life. In sharing their wisdom, Dr. Barke and Dr. Geehr invite the reader to join them in their mission of protecting children from the corrupt, money-driven vaccine industry and honor a view of healthcare based on the principles of truth, knowledge, and medical freedom."

—Dr. Shannon Kroner, author of *I'm Unvaccinated and That's Ok!* and executive director of Freedom Of Religion-United Solutions

"[*Unavoidably Unsafe*] is of . . . critical import at this time in history. People have lost faith that their government—and even their own doctors—can be trusted as reliable sources of medical and scientific information. This book fills a vital role for parents who have become concerned about the safety of all vaccines. It is chock-full of immediately practicable material. It's perfect for busy parents who want a thorough, but readable, reference on vaccines."

—Christopher Rake, MD, MPH

Unavoidably Unsafe

Unavoidably Unsafe

CHILDHOOD VACCINES RECONSIDERED

Edward Geehr, MD
and
Jeffrey Barke, MD

Foreword by Del Bigtree

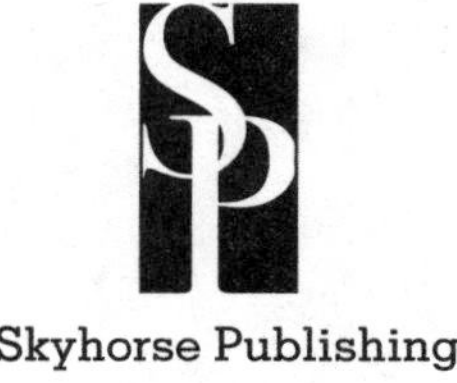

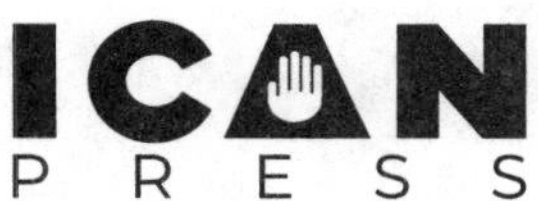

Disclaimer: This book does not offer medical advice and should be considered for educational purposes only. The information contained herein has not been approved by the FDA and should not be used for the diagnosis, treatment, or prevention of any health condition or disease. The content of this book challenges conventional wisdom regarding vaccines. Consequently, it takes courage and patience on the part of the reader to consider and understand the arguments presented. Significant effort has been made to provide supporting documentation and citations. All scientific articles are subject to interpretation and the views expressed in the book may contradict the opinions of those authors and statements by the FDA, CDC, and NIH. Such is the scientific method. Please consult your healthcare provider before acting on any information that may be contained in this book.

Skyhorse Publishing books may be purchased in bulk at special discounts for sales promotion, corporate gifts, fund-raising, or educational purposes. Special editions can also be created to specifications. For details, contact the Special Sales Department, Skyhorse Publishing, 307 West 36th Street, 11th Floor, New York, NY 10018 or info@skyhorsepublishing.com.

Visit our website at www.skyhorsepublishing.com.

Please follow our publisher Tony Lyons on Instagram @tonylyonsisuncertain.

10 9 8 7 6 5 4 3 2 1

Library of Congress Cataloging-in-Publication Data is available on file.

Cover design by Brian Peterson

Print ISBN: 978-1-64821-096-9
Ebook ISBN: 978-1-64821-097-6

Printed in the United States of America

This book is dedicated to JT, who encouraged me to discover the truth about vaccines, and to our grandchildren and their parents, who are confronted with a confusing array of vaccine choices but have lacked the information to empower true informed consent.

—Edward Geehr, MD

This book is dedicated to the millions of children and their parents and guardians who are confused and concerned about the proliferation of childhood vaccines and reports of vaccine injuries. The public is poorly informed about the risks and benefits of vaccines, making proper informed consent nearly impossible. Despite all the advances of modern medicine and a growing list of vaccines, our children are less healthy than ever. There is an epidemic of illness in our children, with 30% being obese. Classrooms are filled with children suffering from food allergies, allergic rhinitis, ADHD, anxiety, gluten sensitivity, peanut allergies, dairy intolerance, and other chronic illnesses. Yet, our government partners with the bio-pharmaceutical industry to keep the vaccine pipeline full of new products, all the while shielding manufacturers from product liability. It is time that our government agencies address and investigate the underlying causes of the declining health of our children. This book intends to shed light on the critical need for proper vaccine informed consent and how parents can become better educated advocates for their children.

—Jeffrey Barke, MD

Contents

Foreword

The first time I saw Dr. Barke was in a viral video on May 9, 2020, in the heart of the COVID pandemic. Wearing dark sunglasses, green doctor's scrubs, and a lab coat, he was speaking at a rally in California, objecting to the insane pandemic policies and making declarative statements like, "Never in the history of this great republic have we quarantined the healthy." For our staff at *The HighWire*, who had been tirelessly battling the storm of mainstream propaganda, it was a ray of sunshine piercing through the dark clouds of global deceit. There was hope.

Though Dr. Barke was one of the first mainstream doctors to speak out against the COVID lockdowns, he certainly wasn't the last. As the experimental COVID vaccine was rushed through the approval process at "Warp Speed," more and more doctors began to wake up to the potential dangers of an mRNA technology that had never been injected into humans. Through the use of alternative media and podcasts, those doctors shared a common warning: "The COVID vaccine isn't as safe as the vaccines we give our kids because it was rushed through safety trials." For most, this was as far as they would allow their pharmaceutical skepticism to take them. But not Dr. Barke or Dr. Geehr. They are two of the few who dared to ask the more important question: "If the CDC is lying about the safety of the COVID vaccine, is it possible that they lied about the safety of all the rest?"

Unavoidably Unsafe takes us on a captivating journey into one of the most dangerous questions any doctor could ask: "Are vaccines safe?" On their quest for the truth, Dr. Barke and Dr. Geehr deftly guide us across the precarious cliffs of vaccine development, over the deep chasms of medical education, to the "Temple of Vaccinia," which, just as it sounds, proves to be much more of a religion than a science.

This book will not be heralded by your doctor, your health department, or even your government. But if you are still holding this book and reading these words, odds are you have already taken a stand. You have chosen to question the mainstream narrative in search of the truth. This book is for those who are willing to wait for the accolades from their own children, who will one day grow up to realize that the reason they are so much healthier than all of their friends and so much more capable than their peers is because their parents were brave enough to abandon the security of consensus, take command of their child's most important health decision, and read this book.

This is the book I have always wanted to write. I am more than proud that our non-profit is involved in making it a success.

Del Bigtree
Host of *The HighWire*
CEO of the Informed Consent Action Network (ICAN)

Preface

> "There is nothing more difficult . . . than to take the lead in the introduction of a new order of things."
>
> —Niccolò Machiavelli, *The Prince*

Few topics in medicine engender more controversy than challenging the wisdom of vaccines. The shots have held a venerated place in the minds of physicians and the lay public alike for decades. As physicians, our vaccine training was nominal, yet we accepted at face value the benefits of vaccines to the public weal as an article of faith. No remedies are more sacrosanct in the halls of medicine.

The intended purpose of vaccines is to allow people to obtain immunity without the risk that comes from getting sick. Their role in taming the great scourge of polio in the 1950s and the global elimination of smallpox in the 1970s is burned into our collective consciousness. Vaccines were universally embraced despite missteps along the way.

Smallpox in the US was already in sharp decline by the 1940s, prior to the introduction of routine vaccination with a standardized, freeze-dried product. The vaccine's ultimate value was eradication of the disease in endemic countries. The early versions of the Salk and Sabin polio vaccines had serious adverse effects, including new cases of polio, necessitating their withdrawal. The latest version still only moderates but does not eradicate infection and transmission.

The Diphtheria, Tetanus, Pertussis (DTP) vaccine was introduced in 1948 and, like the smallpox and polio vaccines, was credited with dramatic reductions in the incidence of hospitalizations and deaths. But similar to the polio vaccines, serious complications attributable to the vaccine necessitated its eventual replacement by the current Diphtheria, Tetanus, acellular Pertussis (DTaP) formulation in 1997.

In fact, it was the avalanche of personal injury litigation arising from DPT vaccine injury that led to the National Childhood Vaccine Injury Act (NCVIA) of 1986, indemnifying the vaccine manufacturers against product liability.

Nevertheless, the promise of vaccines as having near-mystical power to prevent disease was firmly established and broadly accepted. The NCVIA opened the vaccine development floodgates. With blanket liability protection and a favorable regulatory environment, manufacturers turned their attention to what was to become a very profitable line of business.

Prior to 1986, there were four vaccines covering eight diseases on the market for children: Smallpox, DPT, Oral Polio Virus (OPV) and Measles, Mumps, Rubella (MMR). Hemophilus influenza type b (Hib) was approved in 1985 but not placed on the recommended immunization schedule until 1989.

By 2010, the Childhood Immunization Schedule expanded to ten vaccines covering fourteen diseases, including DTaP, MMR, Inactivated Polio Virus (IPV), Hib, Hepatitis B, Varicella (Chickenpox), Hepatitis A, Pneumococcal, Influenza and Rotavirus.

The 2024 Schedule includes the 2010 Schedule, plus Respiratory Syncytial Virus (RSV), COVID-19, and Meningococcal vaccines. By the time an American child reaches twelve months of age they will receive twenty-eight vaccines, beginning the day of their birth, the most of any country. As many as eight vaccines may be given during a single "well child" appointment.

Perhaps more than any other factors, the declining health of children over the past twenty years and the rushed approval and widespread (and often compelled) use of COVID-19 vaccines led us to reevaluate the belief in vaccines we had held so dear. We largely understood the benefits but had limited comprehension of the risks.

As will be discussed in our book, the health of American children is in decline, despite a record number of vaccinations. We will explore the possible contribution of some vaccines to the deteriorating health of our kids.

The COVID-19 vaccines led us and many other physicians (though not enough) to take another look at the vaccine approval process. We were alarmed by the cozy relationship between the FDA and vaccine manufacturers and how Emergency Use Authorization (EUA) shortcut safety studies and informed consent. Equally troubling were the lack of randomized controlled clinical trials proving the safety and effectiveness of common vaccines, and the inclusion of inadequately tested chemicals (called excipients) that have been associated with devastating vaccine complications.

Why Read This Book?

Several excellent books challenge the safety and effectiveness of vaccines. We break new ground and describe:

- The six riskiest childhood vaccines to be eliminated or postponed.
- How the NCVIA undermines the safety of vaccines.
- The revolving door between the pharmaceutical industry and federal regulators.
- Which vaccine approval standards are lower than for drugs.
- How EUA dangerously shortcuts the vaccine approval process.
- Toxic compounds added to vaccines and how they impact developing brains and immune systems.

- The fallacy behind CDC's claim that vaccines do not cause autism.
- Why children should never, ever receive an mRNA vaccine.
- A simple way to score the balance of risks versus benefits of a vaccine for your child.
- The risks to mother and child of the four vaccines recommended during pregnancy.
- Five questions to ask your vaccine provider.
- How to read a vaccine package insert and what to ask your vaccine provider about the contents.
- How to obtain proper informed consent prior to vaccination.
- State-by-state school vaccine exemptions.

Our goal is not to create anti-vaxxers, but to inform vaccine skeptics by arming parents and guardians with information necessary to evaluate the risks and benefits of a vaccine for their child. We are not advising for or against vaccination. Rather, we are fulfilling our professional obligation to ensure patients obtain proper informed consent.

The practice of medicine is based on an imprecise science undergoing constant change. Vaccines are no different. They deserve neither more nor less scrutiny than other aspects of medical care. This book reflects our best effort to update the public and providers alike with the latest.

PROLOGUE

Vaccine Industry and the Revolving Door

> "A revolving door between government and industry can render government agencies more vulnerable to regulatory capture [undue influence]. Both exits to and entries from industry pose a problem for regulatory agencies such as the Department of Health and Human Services."[1]
> —Genevieve Kanter, PhD, associate professor, USC Price School of Public Policy

FDA, Pfizer, & Dr. Gottlieb

The FDA is responsible for protecting public health by ensuring the safety, efficacy, and security of human and veterinary drugs, biologicals, medical devices, the nation's food supply, and vaccines.

Dr. Scott Gottlieb served as FDA Commissioner from May 2017 to April 2019. Midway through Dr. Gottlieb's term, on January 1, 2018, his agency proposed a change to federal regulations governing inspection of facilities licensed to manufacture vaccines and other biological products:

> The Food and Drug Administration . . . is proposing to amend the general biologics regulations relating to time of inspection requirements and also removing duties of inspector requirements. FDA is proposing this action to remove outdated requirements and accommodate new approaches.[2]

Specifically, the rule the FDA wished to change was:

> An inspection of each licensed establishment and its additional location(s) shall be made at least once every 2 years. Inspections may be made with or without notice and shall be made during regular business hours unless otherwise directed.[3]

Changes to inspection requirements for the nation's vaccine suppliers should raise many red flags. During the public comment period, one commenter expressed concern that "the risk-based inspection frequency will not be without negative health consequences," and that "management and mitigation of risk without FDA oversight for a number of years is going to be a high-risk endeavor."[4]

High-risk, indeed. Commissioner Gottlieb's FDA, however, was unmoved, responding:

> We disagree that the risk-based inspection frequency will have negative health consequences.[5]

End of discussion.

On April 2, 2019, just three days before Dr. Gottlieb's last day as Commissioner, the FDA announced that effective May 2, 2019, inspection of licensed facilities (including vaccine manufacturers) would be changed from at least every two years to an indeterminate "risk-based schedule," without defining what "risk-based schedule" means.

Beginning on May 2, 2019, the legal mechanisms through which the FDA regulates vaccine manufacturing virtually disappeared. There was no longer any requirement for FDA inspections, no legal consequences for compliance failures, and inspection of licensed facilities was left entirely to FDA's discretion.[6]

"No Idea" What's Next

In an interview on March 28, 2019, shortly before his departure, Commissioner Gottlieb stated he had "no idea" what he would do next other than spend time with his three young daughters.[7]

Less than three months after Dr. Gottlieb's departure from the FDA, he had an idea about what else he might do with his time. On June 27, 2019, Dr. Gottlieb was elected to Pfizer Inc.'s Board of Directors and was appointed to the board's Regulatory and Compliance Committee. In 2022, Dr. Gottlieb was the highest paid non-executive Pfizer Inc. board member at an annual salary of $553,645.[8]

Following Dr. Gottlieb's appointment to the Pfizer board, three remarkable and unprecedented events occurred in short order.

The first was FDA's authorization (December 11, 2020) of Pfizer-BioNTech COVID-19 vaccine under Emergency Use Authorization (EUA) in individuals sixteen years of age and older (subsequently lowered to just six months of age).[9] Never before had a commercial vaccine, much less one with a completely novel technology, been produced and authorized in less than a year.

The second was the remarkable speed with which Pfizer was able to ramp up production of their newly authorized COVID-19 vaccine to produce millions of vials for worldwide distribution. The company boasted in a 2021 article, "The Shot of a Lifetime":

> How Two Pfizer Manufacturing Plants Upscaled to Produce the COVID-19 Vaccine in ***Record Time***" (emphasis ours).[10]

The third was Pfizer's announcement of record sales of $36.8 billion for its COVID-19 vaccine in 2021 and $37.8 billion a year later, setting pharmaceutical annual sales records for a single product.[11]

It can certainly be argued that Dr. Gottlieb's election to Pfizer's Board of Directors may have been the most consequential appointment in the history of the pharmaceutical industry, or any company for that matter.

A remarkable turnaround for a company that just a few years before (2009) had agreed to pay a $2.3 billion fine, which, according to the US Department of Justice, was the largest fraud settlement in the department's history and the largest criminal fine ever.[12]

CDC, Merck, & Dr. Gerberding

Dr. Julie Gerberding served as Director of the Center for Disease Control (CDC) from 2002 to 2009. According to its website:

> The CDC serves as the national focus for developing and applying disease prevention and control, environmental health, and health promotion and health education activities designed to improve the health of the people of the United States.[13]

As such, the CDC decides which vaccines are going to be placed on the Childhood Immunization Schedule and is tasked with promoting the use of those vaccines for children across the country.

In December 2009, the year Dr. Gerberding stepped down as Director of the CDC, she became president of Merck's vaccine division. During Gerberding's 20 years at Merck, sales in their vaccine division grew from around $1 billion in 2002 to $9.93 billion in 2022, including the blockbuster drug Gardasil®9 ($6.8 B).[14]

Along with GSK, Merck is one of the top two manufacturers of pediatric vaccines including:

- Gardasil®9 for human papilloma virus (HPV)
- M-M-R®II for measles, mumps, and rubella
- Pedvax HIB® for Haemophilus influenzae
- ProQuad® for MMR plus varicella
- RECOMBIVAX HB® for HepB
- RotaTeq® for rotavirus
- VAQTA® for HepA
- VAXNEUVANCE® for pneumococcus
- VAXELIS® for DTaP, Hib, and HepB

Dr. Gerberding retired from Merck in 2022 to become CEO of the Foundation for the National Institutes of Health. The foundation facilitates the very essence of the revolving door, creating and managing alliances between the public and private sectors. The largest foundation donor? The Bill and Melinda Gates Foundation.

The List Goes On

Ten out of eleven of the last FDA commissioners have gone on to work for pharmaceutical companies.[15] The latest, Dr. Stephen Hahn, was FDA commissioner during the COVID-19 crisis, from December 2019 to January 2021. He then joined the biotech investment firm Flagship, the venture fund that launched Moderna, the very company whose COVID-19 vaccine Hahn approved six months before.

The Revolving Door Challenge

The revolving door concept is not unique to the US Department of Health and Human Services (HHS). Other agencies, notably the Departments of Defense, Justice, and Treasury are emblematic of the practice. But HHS leads the pack in people both coming into the department from industry *and* leaving the department to join industry.

Fifteen percent of HHS appointees come from industry, and 32% of those who leave HHS join industry. At the CDC, a division of HHS, only 8% of appointees came from industry–but a whopping 54% left for industry positions.[16]

The revolving door poses an enormous challenge to agencies like the FDA and CDC, guardians of public health in matters of vaccine safety and effectiveness. Pro-industry bias remains a concern while federal regulators flow to and from the industry they regulate. Drs. Gottlieb, Gerberding, and Hahn are just the tip of a very large conflict-of-interest iceberg.

The Focus of This Book

Our greatest concern is the protection of the immune, neurological, and other body systems during a child's most vulnerable, formative years. Consequently, this book focuses on the risks and benefits of each of the twelve vaccines included on the Childhood Immunization Schedule for healthy children up to six years of age. Each vaccine is scored on eight key criteria and assigned an overall rating.

Some discussion is included about children who might disproportionately benefit from vaccination due to underlying illness or therapy, but a full discussion of that topic is beyond the scope of this book.

The burden is not on critics to prove the FDA and CDC wrong but for the agencies to prove that vaccines are safe and effective. They have largely failed in this regard. This book will demonstrate how weak the science behind vaccines included in CDC's Childhood Immunization Schedule really is.

PART ONE

Cracks in the Edifice

CHAPTER 1

The Concept of Unavoidably Unsafe

> "The thing that bugs me is that the people think the FDA is protecting them. It isn't. What the FDA is doing and what the public thinks it's doing are as different as night and day."
>
> —Herbert Lay, MD, former FDA Commissioner[1]

Vaccine Manufacturers Escape Liability

In 1916, a polio epidemic in New York City infected several thousand people leading to 2,000+ deaths. Most of these were children, and death came quickly once the disease took hold. In a study of fatal cases, 82% died within the first week.[2] Many of those who didn't die were left with lifelong disabilities.[3]

Later, in the 1950s, summer polio outbreaks in the US caused tens of thousands of cases, this time leaving hundreds paralyzed or dead. The government was under enormous pressure to develop and deploy a vaccine to fight the recurring epidemics that struck fear across the nation.

It was within this context that the announcement of a polio vaccine, developed by Dr. Jonas Salk in April 1955, was received with great fanfare.

"Safe, effective, and potent." This is how Dr. Thomas Francis, Director of the Poliomyelitis Vaccine Evaluation Center at the University of Michigan, described the results of polio vaccine field trials on more than 1.8 million children. The Salk vaccine, a killed virus vaccine produced by treating live virus with formaldehyde, was up to 90% effective in preventing paralytic polio.[4]

As the nation celebrated this remarkable achievement, pressure was building on the government to ramp up production and disseminate the new vaccine across the country.

Several pharmaceutical companies were given licenses to make the vaccine, including Cutter Laboratories, in Berkeley, California. Cutter went all out, producing and shipping vaccine doses as fast as they could–you might even say at "warp speed."

Tragically, Cutter lost control of its manufacturing process in its haste to meet the demand. The method used to inactivate the live virus proved to be defective. Around 120,000 doses of Cutter's vaccine containing live polio virus were distributed in five western and midwestern states. Within days, there were reports of paralysis among the newly vaccinated. Forty thousand cases of polio were recorded, leaving two hundred children paralyzed and ten dead.

Within a month, the polio mass vaccination program was shut down.

The Salk vaccine was replaced by Sabin's oral, live attenuated polio vaccine (OPV), which meant the live virus was altered so that it wouldn't (theoretically) replicate in the nervous system of humans but could still confer immunity. Given orally, Sabin's vaccine was easier to administer (usually in the form of a sugar cube) than Salk's injectable vaccine and contributed to widespread immunity and a sharp decline in polio cases.[5]

Unfortunately, Sabine's OPV also resulted in the transmission of polio to vaccine recipients, albeit at a much lower rate than with the Salk vaccine. Polio transmission from the OPV continued into the eighties and nineties at a rate of one per 500,000 vaccinations per year until a new inactivated poliovirus (IPV) was approved for use in the US in 2000.[6]

The Cutter Incident

In what came to be known as the Cutter Incident, a number of lawsuits were filed against family-owned Cutter Laboratories, resulting in an award of significant monetary damages. This opened the floodgates, and three more vaccine manufacturers were sued, settling the cases out of court.[7]

The Cutter Incident was followed in 1976 by government overreaction to fears of a swine flu pandemic. A swine flu outbreak among soldiers at Fort Dix led to a mass vaccination campaign where 48 million people were vaccinated in ten months, far more than necessary to control any potential spread.[8]

Cases of Guillain-Barré syndrome, a neurologic condition characterized by progressive weakness and paralysis, began to crop up in swine flu vaccine recipients in excess of what might be expected. In response to these adverse events, government officials shut down the swine flu vaccination program.[9]

Around this same time, the DTP vaccine (diphtheria, tetanus, and pertussis) was implicated in childhood disabilities and developmental delays. This was followed by a sharp rise in vaccine injury tort litigation (an act or omission that gives rise to injury or harm to another).[10]

Generally regarded as a low margin business, vaccine manufacturing was considered by many in the public health community to be at risk of suffering unsustainable financial losses due to vaccine injury litigation, putting further vaccine development at risk.

Although government-industry collaborations were a common thread in these problematic mass vaccination programs, the government response was to look for a mechanism to extend even greater control over the process. After all, if a little bit of government intrusion isn't working, why not try *a lot* more?

In 1983, the National Institutes of Health formed The Committee on Public-Private Sector Relations in Vaccine Innovation.[11] The Committee's purpose was as follows:

> The Committee on Public-Private Sector Relations in Vaccine Innovation was established on the premise that maintaining and extending the control of infectious diseases through immunization is an important national health objective. In compliance with its charge, it undertook a comprehensive study of vaccine research and development, production and supply, and utilization. It paid particular attention to the institutional arrangements and interactions required to ensure vaccine availability and use, and reviewed previous efforts to identify and resolve problems in these areas.[12]

The government was now in the vaccine business as both regulator and promoter, in league with private industry. It would serve as a regulator through FDA vaccine approvals and also a partner in vaccine promotion through the CDC.

In a recommendation that was to become one of the *greatest concessions to US private industry in history*, the Committee advocated a shift in vaccine liability from the manufacturers to the government (Vaccine Injury Compensation and Liability Remedies) and ultimately to the taxpayers.[13]

In other words, *privatize the profits and federalize the liabilities.*

But how can one rationalize such an unprecedented transfer of risk?

Unavoidably Unsafe

The toxicity of vaccines was so well established that exemption from liability was based on the theory that vaccines are **unavoidably unsafe**[14] products, a concept that was adopted by the Supreme Court in the landmark case Bruesewitz v. Wyeth LLC.[15,16]

In addition to federal assumption of liability for all vaccine-related industry, the Committee recommended:[17]

- Supplementary (non-exclusive) compensation system
- Compensation system with restricted tort options
- Mandatory claim review by a compensation board with tort option
- Supplementary compensation system and a vaccine supply public insurance program
- Vaccine supply public insurance program and promotion of no-fault insurance for vaccine-related injury
- Changes in the tort law relating to liability for vaccine-related injury
- Acceptance of vaccine price increases to cover liability costs

As a result of the Committee report, The National Childhood Vaccine Injury Act (NCVIA) was passed by Congress in 1986 to specifically exempt vaccine manufacturers from product liability based on the legal principle that vaccines are unavoidably unsafe products.

However, there was one great caveat attached to the concept of unavoidably unsafe, which has been observed more in the breach than the observance since it was recommended by the NIH in 1985:

> [A]manufacturer will be liable if he markets a drug or vaccine with known risks and fails to warn of them, and it can be shown that the recipient would not have taken the drug or vaccine had he known of the risks.[18]

As will be shown in this book, efforts to inform the public about the risks of vaccines have been so watered down that discussion of risks prior to vaccination, either by health-care providers or through CDC Vaccine Information Statements, have become superficial and cursory.[19]

> Unavoidably unsafe means that even when properly prepared, it is not possible to make a completely safe product and that potential risks of a product are outweighed by its benefits to an individual and society as a whole (subject to a number of conditions under tort law beyond the scope of this book).

Rather than letting market forces and threats of litigation pressure vaccine manufacturers to make a safer product, the government set out to insulate the industry instead. Unavoidably unsafe was to become safe and effective by Congressional declaration, at least as far as vaccine manufacturers were concerned.

Moreover, the government agreed to price increases, subsidies, and to help with vaccine promotion. One need only look at the enormous sums the CDC has been allocating to promote vaccination in children and adults to see just how invested they are.

For example, in 2021, over $3 billion in funding was allocated to states, localities, and jurisdictions through the existing CDC Immunization and Vaccines for Children cooperative agreement.[20]

According to a CDC press release on January 6, 2021:

> Over $3 billion will be made available in an initial award to jurisdictions through the existing CDC Immunization and Vaccines for Children cooperative agreement. These awards will support a range of COVID-19 vaccination activities across jurisdictions. In 2022, CDC spent $680 million to promote childhood vaccines.[21]

That's a lot of marketing dollars the vaccine manufacturers don't have to spend that can fall to their bottom line. Free marketing and no liability risk–what's not to like?

Full Speed Ahead

Given the green light, vaccine production ramped up dramatically, as has the Childhood Immunization Schedule. It makes perfect sense. If a company has no liability for the products they make, and the government is going to subsidize and promote the products, then full speed ahead.

In 1983, three years before the passage of the NCVIA, the Childhood Immunization Schedule included eleven doses of four vaccines. As of early 2024, the number of vaccines on the CDC-recommended childhood schedule has ballooned to eighty-nine doses of seventeen vaccines.[22] American infants receive more vaccines in their first year than infants anywhere in the world: DTaP (3), IPV (3), Hib (3), HepB (3), PCV (4), RV (3), Flu (2), C-19 (2), RSV (2).[23]

Access the full CDC Childhood Immunization Schedule via the below QR code:

Legal Challenges

In 2011, the NCVIA was upheld by the Supreme Court as constitutional in the case of BRUESEWITZ *v.* WYETH, LLC. However, the dissenting opinion by Justice Sotomayor cut to the heart of the decision. She pointed out the potential consequences of removing accountability from vaccine makers. The dissent read, in part,

> Neither the FDA nor any other federal agency, nor state and federal juries—ensures that vaccine manufacturers adequately take account of scientific and technological advancements. This concern is especially acute with respect to vaccines that have already been released and marketed to the public. Manufacturers, *given the lack of robust competition in the vaccine market, will often have little or no incentive to improve the designs of vaccines that are already generating significant profit margins"* emphasis ours.[24]

Little or no incentive indeed, and the money keeps rolling into the vaccine manufacturers in record amounts.[25] But at what cost to the public?

Questions That Demand Answers

In the course of a lifetime, vaccinations escalated dramatically, due in large part to the well-intended NCVIA. But has the rapid expansion of the Childhood Immunization Schedule following passage of the NCVIA been a good thing, a net benefit to society? And at what price in terms of vaccine injury and death?

CHAPTER 2

First, Do No Harm

"In addition to distorting the research agenda, there is overwhelming evidence that drug-company influence biases the research itself."[1]

—Marcia Angell, MD, former editor-in-chief, *The New England Journal of Medicine*

A fundamental tenet of medical practice is to first, do no harm. This requires careful evaluation of the risks imposed by medical interventions like surgery, therapy, medication–and vaccines. Balancing these risks against potential benefits is key to making informed and safe decisions about your family's health and well-being.

When it comes to vaccines, especially those being given to millions of children, it is imperative that the benefits *substantially* outweigh the risks. At their core, all childhood vaccines should be safe, effective, and necessary. As you'll see, that's not always the case.

Can Childhood Vaccines Cause Harm?

Yes. Nearly all medical interventions can cause harm, and childhood vaccines are no exception. What we are specifically concerned with herein is the magnitude of the risk in relation to the benefits of a given childhood vaccine in the context of individual children and society at large (i.e., healthy immune systems, herd immunity, etc.).

The benefits can be considerable, but the risks are notable too.

Hepatitis vaccine:

- *Prevents transmission of a dangerous virus from an infected mother to child* . . . however,
- Fewer than one in 300 babies are born to hepatitis carriers who can be tested for the infection, so should every child bear the inflammatory risks of that vaccine in their first twenty-four hours of life?

MMR vaccine:

- *Protects the vulnerable fetus from congenital rubella syndrome* . . . however,
- MMR vaccine is associated with numerous nervous and immune system disorders.

DTaP vaccine:

- *DTaP blocks the effects of diphtheria's damaging exotoxin* . . . however,
- Diphtheria is extremely rare in the US and excellent treatments are available.
- DTaP vaccine contains aluminum salts plus other known toxins including formaldehyde and Polysorbate 80.
- Four doses are given before one year of age.

Given the totality of these key points, is it safe to say all childhood vaccines do more good than they do harm? All the above with the added risk of post-vaccination symptoms like swelling, vomiting, and (less commonly) seizures or fevers of 105°F and higher, suggests not.[2]

Children's health care should always be grounded in safety, an ideal you'll see is a focal point within the chapters that follow. According to the FDA, Code of Federal Regulations, Title 21:

> The word safety means the relative freedom from harmful effect . . . taking into consideration the character of the product in relation to the condition of the recipient at the time.[3]

The Childhood Vaccine Schedule: There Was No Plan

Most imagine the seventeen recommended childhood vaccines are the result of a well thought out strategy to protect children. That's not the case. The Childhood Immunization Schedule was developed bit-by-bit over time, right alongside the approval of new vaccines.

Each new vaccine that is approved for the schedule has the potential to return $1 billion or more in annual revenue. This is a strong incentive for all shareholders to A) keep producing vaccines for children and B) turn a blind eye to the lack of product liability and overly compliant FDA/CDC regulators.

The evidence? According to the World Council of Health, "[t]he number of vaccines given to babies and children has increased dramatically without the necessary due diligence by regulatory authorities. Parents are urged to adopt a common-sense, 'Safer to Wait' approach.[4]

Childhood vaccines should be evaluated as distinct, complex biochemical systems with unique safety and risk/benefit profiles. These profiles should incorporate insights relevant to age at vaccination, health status of the child, and how rigorously each vaccine is tested for both safety and effectiveness.

CDC Alters the Definition of Vaccine

This inevitably affects the risk-benefit assessment of vaccines—as they become less about protection and more about getting an immune response, the risk-benefit calculation must shift.

Until 2015, the CDC held that vaccination was intended to prevent disease. Most people still perceive vaccination in this manner. Prior to 2015, CDC defined vaccination as, "Injection of a killed or weakened infectious organism in order to prevent disease."[5]

After 2015, there was a subtle change in the definition of a vaccine. The CDC defined a vaccine as "a product that stimulates a person's immune system to produce immunity to a specific disease, protecting the person from that disease."[6]

Then on September 1, 2021, the definition was altered once again. A vaccine was now defined by the CDC as, "A preparation that is used to stimulate the body's immune response against diseases."[7]

Consider that the definition of vaccine migrated in a few short years from disease prevention, to produce immunity to a disease, to stimulate an immune response. Why would the CDC make this change?

As will be discussed, FDA vaccine approvals and CDC vaccine recommendations have increasingly relied on the demonstration of a vaccine-induced immune response rather than evidence of disease prevention. Importantly, the two are not the same. Increases in antibodies following vaccination to particular viruses or bacteria do not mean that the disease will be prevented or lessened.

The change in definition was especially important for the COVID-19 vaccines, as none of the vaccines were studied for disease prevention in children under twelve. They were only tested for antibody responses.

The altered definition also changes the risk-benefit calculus. A vaccine that prevents disease offers greater benefit compared to risks than does a vaccine that only stimulates an immune response.

Excipients: Vaccine Ingredients

Many vaccines contain excipients (ingredients) including adjuvants, preservatives, and stabilizers like aluminum salts,[8] emulsions, and lipids. Adjuvants are included to stimulate a robust immune response to the vaccine's antigens. Vaccine antigens are weakened or inactive parts of target viruses.[9]

Vaccines may also contain contaminants from the manufacturing process, the most recent and egregious example of which is the contamination of COVID-19 mRNA vaccines by plasmid DNA and segments of Simian Virus 40 (SV40), a known cancer promoter.[10]

Aluminum Toxicity

Aluminum phosphate is an adjuvant found in multiple pediatric vaccines, including diphtheria, tetanus, and hepatitis. It is used to boost antibody response since injected aluminum compounds are well-absorbed.

Here's how it works: aluminum-containing vaccines are injected deep into the muscle, and the aluminum ions dissolve and damage surrounding tissues. In turn, the damaged cells release chemical signals that summon immune cells to the area. The subsequent inflammation caused by the adjuvant enhances the immune response to the vaccine antigens found at the injection site.[11]

Lymphatic drainage of vaccinated tissue may spread the aluminum adjuvant to remote areas of the body.[12] It can even cross the blood-brain barrier and accumulate in the brain.[13]

While aluminum compounds can be an effective adjuvant, they are also known neurotoxins.[14,15] The metal is especially harmful to the brain and nerves and has been implicated in diseases like Alzheimer's,[16] autism,[17] and multiple sclerosis.[18]

Administration of multiple vaccines containing aluminum adjuvants adds a significant toxic burden to a child's developing nervous and immune systems.[19] Injection of 20 vaccines containing around 0.5 milligrams (mg) of aluminum adjuvants each is reportedly the equivalent of consuming over 4,000 mg per day of dietary aluminum. Normal dietary intake of aluminum compounds in children is 2-6 mg per day.[20]

Here's a comprehensive list of vaccines that contain aluminum, as per the CDC:[21]

DTaP & Combination Vaccines with DtaP

- DTaP (Daptacel®), DTaP (Infanrix®), DTaP-HepB-IPV (Pediarix®), DTaP-IPV (Kinrix®), DTaP-IPV (Quadracel®), DTaP –IPV/Hib (Pentacel®), DTaP-IPV-Hib-HepB (VAXELIS®)

Hepatitis A & B Vaccines

- HepA (Havrix®), HepA (Vaqta®), HepB (Engerix-B®), HepB (PREHEVBRIO®), HepB (Recombivax®), HepA/HepB (Twinrix®)

Other Vaccines

- HIB (PedvaxHIB®), HPV (Gardasil®9), MenB (Bexsero®, Trumenba®), Pneumococcal (Prevnar 13®, Prevnar 20®, VAXNEUVANCE®), Td (Tenivac®), Td (Mass Biologics), Td (no trade name), Tdap (Adacel®), Tdap (Boostrix®)

Specific Concerns: Aluminum and Autoimmune Disorders

Aluminum compounds including amorphous aluminum hydroxyphosphate (AAHS), aluminum hydroxide, aluminum phosphate, and potassium aluminum phosphate (Alum) are the most studied and widely used adjuvants.[22] They are powerful immune system activators and, combined with vaccine antigens, are said to boost antibody responses up to 100-fold.[23] There may, however, be a price to pay for using such powerful adjuvants.

The term "autoimmunity" is used to describe what happens when the body's immune system begins attacking its own cells as if they were foreign invaders. Several research reports suggest that autoimmunity may be triggered by vaccine adjuvants.[24] Specifically, extreme provocation of the immune system by aluminum compounds may cause the immune system to attack tissue proteins with similar structure to vaccine antigens. Shoenfeld's syndrome is one example of a recognized autoimmune/inflammatory syndrome induced by adjuvants, commonly referred to as ASIA.

Symptoms of ASIA resemble those of other autoimmune diseases and include muscle and joint aches, chronic fatigue, and dry mouth. ASIA-related neurological signs include cognitive disturbances, memory loss, and neurologic disabilities similar to Guillain-Barré Syndrome.[25]

Aluminum and Asthma

Aluminum adjuvants may play a role in the development of asthma as well. A 2023 study led by Kaiser Permanente's Institute for Health Research in collaboration with the CDC found an association between aluminum exposure from vaccines administered before age 24 months and persistent asthma at age 24-59 months.[26]

Aluminum Content Varies Widely in Vaccines

Given the protean toxic effects of aluminum on the body, it behooves the pharmaceutical industry to maintain tight manufacturing controls over aluminum content to assure vaccine safety.

Sadly, this doesn't seem to be the standard.

A 2022 study that measured the amount of aluminum content in infant vaccines found that *only three of thirteen vaccines contained the amount of aluminum indicated by the manufacture*r.[27] Six vaccines contained significantly more aluminum than stated on the package insert. Notably, aluminum content measured in one hepatitis vaccine varied by 350% between lots.[28]

When the researchers who conducted the aluminum content study queried the FDA about who is responsible for verifying aluminum content in vaccines, they uncovered a disturbing answer. The FDA relies fully on data provided by manufacturers–who use unspecified methods–and, even worse, this data is not publicly available.[29]

Even though FDA approval for vaccines should be extremely rigorous and transparent to assure the public of vaccine safety and effectiveness, the process relies on manufacturers' good faith.

Are Aluminum Compounds Found in Pediatric Vaccines Safe?

There is no direct answer when it comes to whether the aluminum compounds in children's vaccines are safe. They have neither consistent manufacturing controls nor a proven safety profile. Moreover, the authors of the aluminum study referenced in the previous section note that a recent FOIA (Freedom of Information Act) request revealed the National Institutes of Health (NIH) was "unable to provide a single study relied upon by them in relation to the safety of injection of aluminum adjuvants in infants."[30] Until convincing evidence is received to the contrary, aluminum adjuvants must be considered as contributing factors to widely documented vaccine adverse events.

Here is a partial list of pediatric vaccine excipients as listed by the CDC,[31] most of which are considered toxic or controversial to some degree:

- Formaldehyde/Formalin (inflammatory, corrosive)
- Beta propiolactone (corrosive, carcinogen)
- Hexadecyltrimethylammonium bromide (corrosive)
- Aluminum hydroxide (inflammatory, neurotoxic)
- Aluminum phosphate (inflammatory, neurotoxic)
- Thimerosal (preservative, removed from vaccines except influenza)
- Polysorbate 80 (hypersensitivity reaction, crosses blood-brain barrier)
- Glutaraldehyde (can be cytotoxic)
- Fetal Bovine Serum (exposure to bovine proteins and disease)
- African Green Monkey Kidney Cells (exposure to SV40)
- Acetone (solvent that may be cytotoxic)
- Human Embryonic Lung Cell Cultures (from aborted fetuses)
- DNA from Porcine Circovirus Type-1 (immune dysregulation)

The vast majority of children receive the full suite of childhood vaccinations by the age of two, which means repeated exposure to toxic excipients like aluminum.[32] Regardless of the presence of various excipients and adjuvants, all childhood vaccines are nevertheless administered as if they are equivalent in terms of safety and efficacy, accepted because they are "on the schedule."

Parents/guardians and providers often blindly follow the Childhood Immunization Schedule, except in cases where a known allergy to an ingredient is present. Outside of these infrequent exceptions, childhood vaccines are broadly accepted and regarded as safe and necessary for the good of society.

High Degree of Variability Between Vaccines

In coming chapters, the high degree of variability between vaccines is demonstrated, including types of antigens selected, immune system response, duration, safety, effectiveness, and reactogenicity. The latter refers to the physical signs of the body's inflammatory response to vaccines such as injection site pain, redness, swelling, and systemic symptoms such as fever, muscle aches, joint pain, or headache.[33]

Childhood vaccines are often "bundled" together. For example, a six-month-old can receive as many as eight injections at a time.[34] Yet, there is limited data about the risks of giving multiple vaccine injections at once. In fact, recent reviews have led to questions about the safety of multiple vaccinations during a single visit.[35,36] The long-term consequences of this practice are unknown, and there is little evidence to support the safety of multiple, simultaneous vaccinations. Some researchers have suggested the potential for biochemical or synergistic toxicity due to multiple vaccines administered concurrently.[37]

Vaccines and Autism

The CDC has made the definitive statement that vaccines do not cause autism.[38] However, there is growing concern about whether vaccines are in fact contributing to observations of increased rates of neurodevelopmental disorders, including autism.[39,40,41,42,43]

What the CDC does not disclose is that none of the first twenty vaccines given to infants have been studied for their relationship to autism. MMR is in fact the *only* vaccine that's been evaluated for links to autism, and it is not given until children are twelve months old. CDC's absolute denial of causation will be shown in Chapter 10, MMR and Autism Spectrum Disorder (ASD)—The Great Debate, to be tenuous at best.[44,45]

Finally, autism diagnoses have risen dramatically since 2000, as shown in the figure below. The data in the chart reflects CDC data that was also part of a press release by The Autism Community in Action (TACA) in March of 2023.[46,47]

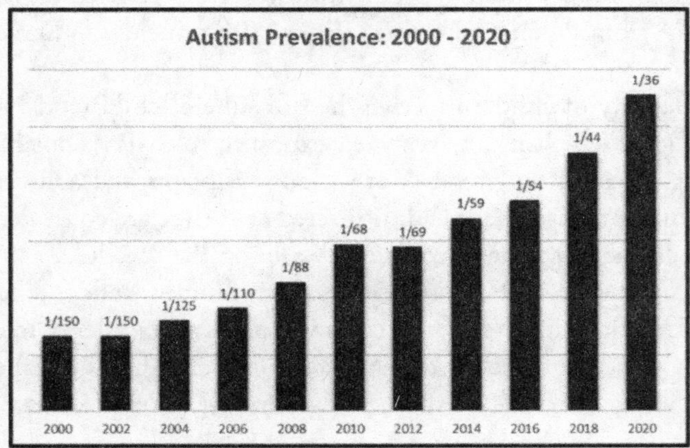

The societal costs of autism are staggering, estimated to be over $500 billion per year in 2030.[48]

Vaccine Risk-Benefit Profile for Individual Children is Poorly Understood

The decision about whether to administer any single vaccine to a specific child must be considered on an individual basis before an informed decision can be made.

All children possess a unique biochemistry and genetic makeup that makes them more or less susceptible to various types of antigens and excipients. Just because one child tolerates vaccination does not mean the next won't suffer a neurodevelopmental disorder as a result of the same vaccine. Similarly, a single vaccine may be well-tolerated whereas multiple simultaneous vaccinations may result in a serious adverse event.

The CDC has issued a Child and Adolescent Immunization Schedule by Medical Indication, Recommendations for Ages 18 or Younger.[49] The schedule makes recommendations regarding withholding, delaying, precautions, contraindications, and additional doses for each of the childhood vaccinations. It considers conditions like pregnancy, immune status, HIV infection, kidney failure, hemodialysis, and diabetes when deciding on vaccine administration.

The Schedule is useful but limited. What is needed is a more detailed and robust understanding of biochemical and genetic factors that may predispose children to serious vaccine adverse events from vaccine components and combinations.

Misleading the Way: A Look Into How Vaccine Manufacturers Calculate Effectiveness

The FDA accepts a lesser standard for calculating and reporting the benefit of vaccines as compared to drugs. Without stretching the truth, we can say that vaccine manufacturers report vaccine effectiveness in a manner that presents their product as favorably as possible, even if it's a bit misleading.

First, it's important to understand the term "risk reduction." It refers to a vaccine or drug's effectiveness in reducing the risk of contracting the condition it was developed to prevent or treat. So, let's say a vaccine's effects were studied in a trial of 2,000 people: 1,000 received the vaccine, and 1,000 were in the control group. Of the 1,000 vaccinated people, 18 got the disease; 61 people in the control group were infected.

Vaccine manufacturers would use something called the Relative Risk Reduction (RRR) calculation to arrive at an impressive 70.5% effectiveness at reducing the likelihood of getting the disease if vaccinated (the formula is here[50]).

What most people don't know is that RRR is representative of the general population as a whole. If you want to know a vaccine's risk reduction for each individual who may be exposed, it's better to use the Absolute Risk Reduction (ARR) calculation, which is the one drug manufacturers use when reporting their results.

The ARR calculation for the example study of 2,000 people is just 4.3%. In other words, vaccination reduces the chances of getting infected by 4.3% for each child, a far cry from the headline 70% effectiveness number the FDA and manufactures like to publicize.

There are other techniques used to confirm the probability and statistical significance of RRR or ARR measures that are beyond the scope of this book. But the magnitude of difference between RRR and ARR results for a particular vaccine may prove useful in assessing individual risk compared with the whole group.

A real-world example of widely discrepant RRR and ARR results can be found in a discussion of Vaccine Safety and Effectiveness under Chapter 4, COVID-19. The widely reported RRR of 95% at preventing infection stands in contrast with an ARR of around 1%. A vaccine that offers a 1% reduction in the likelihood of getting infected may not offer a compelling reason to vaccinate in comparison with potential risks.

Being Resourceful: Maternal Antibodies

Antibodies are transferred from mother to child and protect newborns and infants during maturation of their immune system. The transfer occurs prior to birth across the placenta and after birth through colostrum and breast milk.[51] Maternal antibodies are very effective in protecting neonates and infants against most infectious diseases.[52] This protection declines over six to twelve months as maternal antibodies wane.

While maternal antibodies do protect infants, they also interfere with a child's immune response to vaccination during the first year. No current vaccine formulation is fully effective in the presence of maternal antibodies. Why, then, are so many vaccines recommended in the first months of life? The recommendation is contrary to studies that have shown a low level of maternal antibody correlates best with vaccination success.[53] This may help to explain why frequent vaccinations are necessary during the first year to achieve adequate antibody levels.[54]

Maternal antibodies that were passively transferred during pregnancy don't completely disappear until twelve months of age, which may represent the optimal time to initiate the Childhood Immunization Schedule.[55]

Of course, the ideal process would be to first measure the child's antibodies before commencing immunizations, but this option is rarely, if ever, offered.

Vaccine Approval Process

Vaccines are considered biologics and are different from most drugs that are chemically synthesized. Biologics represent a wide range of products, including those derived directly from living organisms or genetically engineered to replicate biological functions. They include vaccines, blood components, gene therapies, and synthesized therapeutic proteins such as hormones, blood clotting factors, and growth factors.

One of the steps in the FDA regulatory approval process, called a Biologics License Application (BLA), subjects all biologics to thorough clinical trials on large numbers of patients, often in the thousands.

Prior to vaccine or biologics approval, there are three phases of clinical trials. The last step (Phase 3), is theoretically a randomized, double-blind, placebo-controlled trial, often known as the gold standard of clinical testing.

For example, the Salk polio vaccine clinical trial enrolled nearly 2 million children in Phase 3 of its trial and lasted just over a year.[56] Despite the trial success, the Cutter Incident cut short the national roll out, as careful oversight of the manufacturing process proved to be just as important as the clinical results.

FDA Standards Fall Short on Childhood Vaccines

Vaccine approvals through a BLA have not been held to the same standard of evidence required of other biologics or of drugs (which follow a separate approval process called a New Drug Application or NDA). **No vaccine** on the CDC's Childhood Immunization Schedule has been subjected to the gold standard of testing: a prospective, randomized, placebo-controlled trial (RCT).

It is critical that an inert placebo, one that has no effect on the immune system, be used in the control group. This ensures the control group is not exposed to substances that might generate side effects, thereby confounding the study results.

For example, according to the Childhood Immunization Schedule, VAXNEUVANCE® is given to infants at ages two, four, six, and twelve months. What did the control group receive during the trial? Not saline, as it turns out, but an earlier generation product, Prevnar 13®. Severe adverse events were nearly equal in both groups.[57]

It cannot be known how safety measures in the VAXNEUVANCE® group would compare with a true, saline-injected control group because there never was one. Nevertheless, the FDA approved the vaccine in 2010, based in part on the lack of a notable safety signal between the new and older versions of the same vaccine; in other words, they were equally risky.

The core argument against an RCT for vaccines is that it is unethical to withhold a vaccine from a control group who are at risk of contracting a disease. It can pit a doctor's therapeutic obligation to offer optimal care to all against undermining the scientific and clinical integrity of an RCT.

However, if the rationale for an RCT is to optimize the scientific validity of a vaccine clinical trial with widespread implications, it is best to get the science right before dissemination to millions of people anyway. On the other hand, putting persons at risk of serious harm as a result of giving them a placebo may violate ethical principles for medical research involving human subjects.[58]

A full discussion of this issue is beyond the scope of this book. However, there are several well-constructed, ethical RCT options available to researchers faced with this dilemma. An excellent discussion of the various RCT options for vaccines can be found within the reference at the end of this sentence.[59]

Chapter 4, COVID-19, includes a discussion of a truncated or even completely skipped clinical trial process that vividly illustrates the disastrous consequences of rushing a vaccine to market.

The fact remains, the lack of a true placebo control group, or in some cases, no control group at all, is the rule and not the exception with every vaccine that appears on the Childhood Immunization Schedule.

Informed Consent

The Nuremberg trials in the aftermath of World War II led to the creation of the Nuremberg Code in 1947. The code stipulates that no person shall be subject to medical experimentation without being fully informed of the risks and benefits, and that they must have the capacity to consent without coercion.

The Nuremberg Code applies to non-experimental medical therapies and treatments (like vaccines) too. Full disclosure of risks and benefits prior to consent, however, is contingent on the quality of clinical trials prior to FDA approval. When these trials are inadequate (as they often are), physicians and parents are left to make decisions in the dark without any real insight into vaccines' risks and benefits.

One of the vaccines on the Childhood Immunization Schedule, the COVID-19 mRNA booster, had no human clinical trials at all prior to receiving an Emergency Use Authorization. The absence of informed consent for these vaccines renders them as medical experimentation, and clearly violates the Nuremberg Code.

The need for informed consent is unquestionable, but controversy prevails over the nature of a truly informed consent. The Belmont Report's "Ethical Principles and Guidelines for the Protection of Human Subjects of Research" contains a useful framework to consider by noting the "widespread agreement that the consent process [has] three elements: information, comprehension and voluntariness."[60]

Recommendations for how parents, guardians, and caregivers can obtain proper informed consent following this framework prior to vaccinating their children will be discussed in Chapter 21, Five Questions to Ask Your Pediatrician.

Vaccines and SIDS

The CDC and the American Academy of Pediatrics state unequivocally that vaccines have not been shown to cause sudden infant death syndrome.[61]

Any observed correlation of the timing and number of vaccines with infant mortality (death) is not necessarily causation. However, the correlation between the timing and number of vaccine doses and SIDS remains the subject of ongoing research.

A 2023 study published in the peer-reviewed journal *Cureus* examined the number of vaccine doses routinely given in developed nations during the neonatal period and infancy and their association with mortality in children at one and five years.[62] In the study, mortality data and vaccine schedules were collected from UNICEF, the World Health Organization (WHO), and various national governments.

Multiple analyses of the available data showed the children who went without any shots did the best. The greater the number of vaccines, the greater the likelihood of neonatal mortality, infant mortality, and under age five mortality. The study authors observed that "[i]n these circumstances health authorities expect to see negative correlations, that is, a decline in mortality with more vaccine doses. So, any statistically significant positive correlation is a genuine concern."[63]

Again, though, this is not proof of causation. This study has a number of limitations based on the data sets used, including the absence of individual child information. Additionally, the exact configuration and causes of death are not specified.

A reasonable interpretation is that less may be more in terms of aggregate number of vaccines administered over a given period of time, further emphasizing advantages of a risk-benefit approach. For example, neonates and infants derive no benefit from HepB vaccine unless they fall under the rare exception of being born to a hepatitis B positive mother, are cared for by hepatitis B carriers, or the infection status of the mother is unknown.

There is no reason a child born to healthy parents and caregivers should routinely receive HepB vaccines. It does not mean that HepB vaccination will necessarily put an infant at risk of SIDS or a neurological disorder, but neither is the risk zero, while the benefit is non-existent for the vast majority of infants.

As will be discussed in greater detail in Chapter 8, DTaP, SIDS has also been linked to DTaP vaccination.

The CDC asserts there is no causal link between childhood vaccines and SIDS yet does not address that the peak age for SIDS is two to four months . . . which coincides with the introduction of thirteen vaccinations during a critical time of growth and development.

More SIDS Correlations: VAERS Data Study

A comprehensive review of existing Vaccine Adverse Event Reporting System (VAERS) data in 2019 found a statistically significant correlation between vaccination and the timing of death.[64] The author examined all infant deaths recorded in VAERS within sixty days of vaccination.

Of the 1,048 SIDS cases identified in the VAERS database, 13% died on the day of vaccination, 51% occurred within three days, and 75% within seven days post-vaccination. The remaining SIDS deaths in the data set occurred between day eight and 60, and 90% of those deaths occurred in infants under six months of age. In a review of 2,605 reported infant deaths from all causes, 58% occurred within three days of vaccination and 78% within seven days of vaccination, *roughly in the same distribution as SIDS deaths.*

Of particular concern is that the rate of SIDS within the first seven days post-vaccination was 57 times the rate of SIDS in days eight to 60, a statistically significant difference.

Argument against Vaccines Causing SIDS

The CDC takes the position that the observed correlations of SIDS and immunizations do not prove that infant deaths were causally related to vaccines. They cite seven research studies and safety reviews that have looked at possible links between vaccines and SIDS. Their findings are that the "evidence accumulated over many years does not show any links between childhood immunization and SIDS."[65,66,67,68,69,70,71]

Careful review of the seven articles cited by the CDC fails to identify definitive evidence to support the CDC's assertion. Each had methodological problems that neither proved nor disproved a causal relationship between vaccination and SIDS. These include:

- A study based on VAERS data that is known to underreport adverse events.
- A discussion of safe sleep environments without any evidence for vaccine safety.
- A study that seemingly contradicts the CDC's position, noting that for child death reports, 79.4% received greater than one vaccine on the same day and 44% of deaths were from SIDS.
- A retrospective cohort study of health plan data without clinical chart review within a highly selected population that may skew the data.
- A systematic review of studies that found data could not rule out an association for several vaccines and admitted the lack of knowledge concerning pathogenesis of SIDS.
- A VAERS study that was equivocal in its findings on whether there might be a causal relationship.
- A study that relied on death certificates without criteria to establish a diagnosis of SIDS and no clinical review of medical records.

Despite the blanket assurance provided by the CDC about the safety of multiple vaccinations during the first year of life, the reports above indicate the relationship between vaccines and SIDS remains unsettled.[72]

Longer-term health risks such as neurodevelopmental disorders, autism, allergies, and asthma also remain far from resolved. The data regarding these issues will be explored in great detail in subsequent chapters.

Are Unvaccinated Children Healthier Than Vaccinated Children?

There is little dispute that the health of American children is in decline. An estimated 43% of US children (32 million) have at least one of twenty chronic health conditions, increasing to 54.1% when adjusted to include children who are overweight, suffer from obesity, or are at risk for developmental delays.[73]

One study that examined this issue was published in 2020 by Hooker and Miller.[74] Their large, peer-reviewed study detailing health outcomes of vaccinated versus unvaccinated children concluded that unvaccinated children have better health outcomes than their vaccinated peers, with fewer cases of asthma, developmental delays, ear infections, and gastrointestinal disorders.[75]

Further research is certainly necessary on this important topic but will require the CDC, NIH, and medical specialty societies to cast aside their biases and take an honest look at the risks of childhood vaccination–perhaps for the first time.

The First Six Vulnerable, Formative Years

This book addresses the Childhood Immunization Schedule for children six years and under. These are formative developmental years when the neurological, immune, cardiovascular, endocrine, GI, and skeletal systems undergo dramatic change and growth.

Brain growth alone is explosive during this period, doubling in size during the first year of life. Synaptic connections between brain cells are made at an astonishing rate: at least one million new neural connections every second.[76]

The injection of foreign proteins and immune system stimulants at this vulnerable stage of life can be highly toxic and disruptive to normal neurodevelopment and other developing organ systems. As such, the goal of this book is to inform parents and providers of the risks and benefits of childhood vaccines. Prior to vaccination, parents and caregivers should consider all factors relevant to a particular child instead of following recommendations based on age alone.

For example, vaccine benefits may outweigh risks for a child whose immune system is compromised by chemotherapy, chronic illness, or an inherited immune disorder. Common childhood illnesses may become life-threatening in immunocompromised children. Moreover, such children may benefit from an increased number and frequency of vaccine doses.

In contrast, children with nervous system disorders or developmental disabilities such as epilepsy, cerebral palsy, autism, muscular dystrophy, and movement disorders may prove to be more susceptible to the toxic effects of such vaccine excipients as aluminum salts, formaldehyde, thimerosal, polysorbate 80 and glutaraldehyde.

Health status, nutrition, living conditions, access to care, family relationships, and attitudes about public health and vaccine mandates are also essential elements of each decision.

Parents of healthy children and their providers must begin leading the effort to assess each vaccine for whether it is safer to wait or eliminate it altogether.[77]

PART TWO

The Risky Six

CHAPTER 3

Meet the Risky Six

"The medical profession is being bought by the pharmaceutical industry . . . The academic institutions of this country are allowing themselves to be the paid agents of the pharmaceutical industry.[1] I think it's disgraceful."

—Arnold Relman, MD, former editor-in-chief, *The New England Journal of Medicine*

There are twelve vaccines on the Childhood Immunization Schedule that are administered by six years of age. Six of these vaccines for children merit special attention. They fail across a number of dimensions, including risks that far outweigh benefits. Moreover, the diseases prevented may be mild, exceedingly rare, or have effective treatments; immunity wanes over time; herd immunity is not established; and risk is elevated for impaired immune function, autoimmune disorders, and neurocognitive disabilities.

The Risky Six include:

- COVID-19
- Hepatitis B
- RSV
- Influenza
- DTaP
- MMR

Criteria for Evaluating Vaccine Safety and Effectiveness

Eight criteria have been selected to thoroughly evaluate the twelve vaccines listed on the Childhood Immunization Schedule that all are typically administered before the age of six years. These criteria draw from components of the CDC's "How Vaccines are Developed and Approved for Use."[2]

1. Children are at high risk of severe illness or death from disease.
2. Vaccine prevents infection and replication.

3. Vaccine prevents transmission to others.
4. Vaccine is approved for use by the FDA.
5. Vaccine safety and efficacy supported by randomized, controlled, clinical trials.
6. Vaccine does not significantly impact developing childhood immune, cardiovascular, neurological, hematological, hormonal, or musculoskeletal systems.
7. Vaccine creates lifelong immunity.
8. Vaccine important to reach herd immunity.

Each vaccine is graded as follows:

Grade	Criteria
A	Evidence is strongly in favor of the criterion.
B	The balance of evidence supports the criterion.
C	There is a roughly equal balance of evidence for and against the criterion.
D	The balance of evidence fails to support the criterion.
F	Evidence strongly opposes the criterion.

Overall Grade as an Indicator of Risks vs. Benefits

Each vaccine is also given an Overall Grade of A-F, based roughly on an average of all grades. The Overall Grade is intended to reflect a balance of a vaccine's risks versus benefits. A higher grade indicates a greater likelihood of benefit, while a lower grade indicates a greater likelihood of risk:

Overall Grade	Explanation
A	Benefits strongly outweigh the risks.
B	Benefits tend to outweigh the risks.
C	Benefits and risks are roughly equivalent.
D	Risks tend to outweigh benefits.
F	Risks strongly outweigh the benefits.

Certain criteria are weighted more heavily than others for some vaccines. For example, a disease that is rare (e.g. diphtheria) or causes mild to no illness in children (e.g. hepatitis A), but with an effective vaccine, will be graded lower than a higher risk disease (e.g. polio) with a less effective vaccine.

Overall grading is intended to serve as one factor parents and guardians can take into consideration when discussing their options with a child's vaccine provider when deciding whether to proceed with the vaccine as scheduled; delay one or more vaccinations; or eliminate one or more vaccinations.

At the beginning of each chapter, you'll find an easy-to-access table that includes a graded assessment of the vaccine being discussed. The Risky Six chapters include detailed discussions of the scored criteria.

Buckle up for the reading ahead. The Risky Six do not inspire confidence in the vaccine approval process.

Why Now? COVID-19 Vaccines Prompt a Closer Look at the Vaccine Schedule

Perhaps more than any other vaccine, the FDA's and CDC's incessant promotion of the COVID-19 vaccine for children calls for a much-needed evaluation of the rest of the Childhood Immunization Schedule.

Despite reassurances from government agencies and the American Academy of Pediatrics, a closer look at the evidence for the safety and effectiveness of the immunization schedule raises more questions than answers. The science behind many vaccine approvals remains incomplete and, in some cases, it's downright misleading.

It may come as a surprise to parents and physicians that *not a single vaccine* listed on the pediatric schedule has been subject to a randomized, controlled clinical trial where the vaccine was compared with a true placebo, such as saline.

Perhaps just as surprising is that unlike drug approvals, FDA vaccine approvals do not require randomized controlled clinical trials against an immunologically inactive placebo. Drugs and vaccines have completely separate approval processes: a New Drug Application (NDA) for drugs and a Biologics License Application (BLA) for vaccines.[3,4]

A major difference between the NDA and BLA processes is that while NDA approval requires comparison with placebos, BLA does not. Instead, BLA approval requires only comparison to other vaccines or biologically active ingredients such as aluminum. This, of course, can obscure the true safety profile of a new vaccine and is a major flaw in the approval process.

Importance of Control Groups During Clinical Trials

Control groups are a critical component of studies and processes aimed at assessing safety. Unfortunately, many pediatric vaccines were approved after being compared to a previous version of the same vaccine–not a neutral control group. Other vaccines' follow-up periods were limited to days/weeks instead of the months to years needed to truly detect safety signals.

> A safety signal is information detected during a clinical trial that may indicate the presence of a serious adverse event potentially caused by a medication or vaccine that warrants further investigation.

For example, the pneumococcal vaccine (PCV15) was tested against a previous version of the same vaccine (PCV13), which was tested against the original vaccine (PCV7), which was tested against an experimental meningococcal vaccine . . . but never against an inert placebo like saline.

Safety signals from the latest vaccine may be obscured by comparison to safety signals from earlier versions, whereas comparison with a placebo with few or no side effects may reveal the true incidence of complications.

The Hepatitis B vaccine (HepB) is an example of inadequate follow-up. HepB, administered the first day of a baby's life, had only four days of safety testing across numerous clinical trials. If a baby in the test group had a serious adverse event after four days, it would not be officially attributed to the vaccine.

Pediatric vaccines EngerixB® (HepB), HAVRIX® (HepA), and Fluarix® (influenza) were never tested for carcinogenesis, mutagenesis (genetic mutations), or impairment of fertility. Yet, they are given to our most vulnerable children whose immature immune systems are undergoing rapid development.

Risks vs. Benefits

As with all medications, vaccines should be evaluated based on their risks and benefits *as applicable to an individual child's health profile.* A decision to vaccinate a child should also be based on informed consent, the exception in most practices, rather than the rule. This is because many practitioners answer questions about vaccines by citing the CDC or American Academy of Pediatrics. Since these sources don't always present the full picture, this is more so an appeal to authority than informed consent.

True informed consent is based on a thorough discussion of risks and benefits, and evidence for each, with respect to your child individually. Chapter 21, Five Questions to Ask Your Pediatrician, discusses how to approach your provider to obtain informed consent.

Possible Risks of vaccination include near and long-term adverse events such as allergic reactions, myocarditis, arrhythmias, neuropsychiatric (ADHD, anxiety) and neurodevelopmental disorders (autism), impaired fertility, cancer, and death (SIDS).

Potential Benefits include decreased incidence of infection and transmission of communicable diseases of significance (high-risk diseases), reduced susceptibility to toxins produced by pathogens (e.g. tetanus, diphtheria), decreased likelihood of cancer due to infectious agents (HPV), and building of herd immunity.

Herd Immunity

The theory of herd immunity holds that individuals at high risk who are unable mount a proper immune response to circulating pathogens naturally or by vaccination will be protected by those around them who have immunity. In effect, those with immunity break or lessen the chain of transmission of infection from one person to another, making it less likely that those at higher risk will become infected.

Herd immunity may be achieved when as few as 50% of the population is immunized or has natural immunity or not until as much as 95% has immunity, depending on the contagiousness of the disease. The more contagious, the higher the percentage necessary for herd immunity.[5]

Persons with healthy immune systems that develop natural immunity through infection and recovery lie at the core of herd immunity. Vaccines can contribute to herd immunity but can never be sufficient by themselves to protect the vulnerable.

That is because thousands of viruses constantly circulate that can infect humans, but there exists a limited number of safe and effective vaccines. Herd immunity will always primarily rely on a healthy population with proper sanitation, clean water, adequate nutrition, shelter, and medical care. Absent those factors, vaccines rarely offer sufficient protection for those who can't mount a proper immune defense themselves. Those at highest risk will always need some measure of additional protection, through restricted visitation, enhanced hygiene, testing of caregivers, or other measures, regardless of how many vaccines are developed.

The Optimal Vaccine

The optimal pediatric vaccine:

- Targets a prevalent, high-risk disease for which limited treatments are available.
- Benefits far exceed the risks.
- Offers an excellent safety profile as demonstrated through long-term, controlled clinical trials containing a true placebo group.
- Is highly effective at preventing infection, replication, and transmission of disease.
- Contributes to herd immunity for highly contagious diseases.
- Does not compromise natural immunity.

Unfortunately, few pediatric vaccines meet all these criteria. The Risky Six vaccines in particular stand out as failing to meet all or most of these optimal criteria for the general pediatric population under six years of age and in good health.

CHAPTER 4

COVID-19

"The best vaccination is to get infected yourself."[1]

—Anthony Fauci, MD

First among the Risky Six vaccines are the COVID-19 mRNA vaccines, FDA authorized for children as young as six months and added to the Childhood Immunization Schedule in 2023.

COVID-19 mRNA vaccines meet none of the criteria that might justify their use.

Criteria	**Grade**
Children are at high risk of severe illness or death from disease	**F**
Vaccine prevents infection and replication	**F**
Vaccine prevents transmission to others	**F**
Vaccine is approved for use by the FDA	**F**
Vaccine safety and efficacy supported by randomized, controlled, clinical trials	**F**
Vaccine does not significantly impact developing childhood immune, cardiovascular, neurological, hematological, hormonal, or musculoskeletal systems	**F**
Vaccine creates lifelong immunity	**F**
Vaccine important to reach herd immunity	**F**
Overall	**F**

The criteria and their respective ratings are discussed below. For additional details, please see Chapter 17, Why You Should Never, Ever Give a Child an mRNA Vaccine.

Vaccine Schedule

The CDC's recommendations for administration of the COVID-19 vaccine are complex. They note that all people 6+ months of age and older should be vaccinated.

Please refer to the CDC's "Interim Clinical Considerations for Use of COVID-19 Vaccines in the United States" via the below QR code to review CDC-recommended COVID-19 vaccine schedules.

Vaccines Offered

Vaccine	Excipients[2]
Comirnaty® (Pfizer-BioNTech)	messenger ribonucleic acid (mRNA), lipids (4-hydroxybutyl) azanediyl)bis(hexane-6,1-diyl)bis(2- hexyldecanoic), 2 [(polyethylene glycol)-2000]-N,N-di tetradecyl acetamide, 1, 2-distearoyl-sn-glycero-3-phosphocholine, and cholesterol), tromethamine, tromethamine hydrochloride, and sucrose. Pfizer-BioNTech COVID-19 Vaccine may also contain sodium chloride
SpikeVAX® (Moderna)	messenger ribonucleic acid (mRNA), lipids (SM-102, polyethylene glycol [PEG] 2000 dimyristoyl glycerol [DMG], cholesterol, and 1,2-distearoyl-sn-glycero-3-phosphocholine [DSPC]), tromethamine, tromethamine hydrochloride, acetic acid, sodium acetate trihydrate, and sucrose
Novavax®	recombinant form of the SARS-CoV-2 Spike protein produced from baculovirus infected Sf9 (fall armyworm) insect cells and MatrixMTM adjuvant containing saponins derived from the soapbark tree (Quillaja saponaria Molina). Other ingredients include cholesterol, phosphatidylcholine, potassium dihydrogen phosphate, potassium chloride, disodium hydrogen phosphate dihydrate, sodium chloride, disodium hydrogen phosphate heptahydrate, sodium dihydrogen phosphate monohydrate, polysorbate 80. The vaccine may also contain small amounts of baculovirus and insect cell proteins and DNA

Contraindications include history of a severe allergic reaction after a previous dose or to a component of the COVID-19 vaccine.[3]

Children at High Risk from Disease—F

- Severe illness and death in children extremely rare
- Many studies report no deaths in healthy children
- Vast majority of children have natural immunity
- Natural immunity effective against Omicron variants

Severe illness and death in a healthy child from COVID-19 is extremely rare.[4,5] The most recent data posted by the American Academy of Pediatrics showed that "[c]hildren were 0.00%-0.19% of all COVID-19 deaths, and 10 [US] states reported zero child deaths."[6]

Several studies have failed to detect a single fatality in a child without comorbidities (underlying chronic health conditions).[7,8] Of note is that these estimates occurred before the emergence of weaker Omicron variants.

The CDC estimates that over 96% of children have now been exposed to COVID-19.[9] Children are known to develop a more powerful binding (blocking) and neutralizing (killing) antibody responses to SARS-CoV-2 infection than adults, conferring robust and enduring immunity.[10] Natural immunity has also proven highly effective at preventing reinfection from Omicron variants.[11,12,13]

Remarkably, the CDC refuses to acknowledge that previous COVID-19 infections provide protective, natural immunity. This is in stark contrast with the CDC's current recommendation that evidence of previous infection with common childhood diseases such as chickenpox, measles, mumps, and rubella precludes the need for vaccination.[14,15]

Vaccine Prevents Infection—F

- COVID-19 vaccines do not prevent infection
- Rapid deterioration of vaccine effectiveness
- More vaccinations correlate with greater risk of infection

COVID-19 vaccines do not prevent infection. A study of nearly 900,000 children aged five to eleven published in the *New England Journal of Medicine* shows that mRNA vaccine effectiveness rapidly deteriorates over a few weeks and becomes negative over time (meaning vaccination actually increases risk of infection).[16]

Another study of 50,000+ employees of the Cleveland Clinic showed the greater the number of vaccinations, the more likely staff were to become infected with COVID-19.[17]

A Danish study had results similar to those of the Cleveland Clinic. After just three months, the vaccine effectiveness of Pfizer and Moderna turned negative. Pfizer recipients were 76.5% more likely and Moderna recipients 39.3% more likely to be infected than unvaxxed people.[18]

The CDC has cautioned that authorized COVID-19 vaccines may not be effective against the latest variants.[19] This should be no surprise, as there has never been a safe and effective vaccine developed to prevent a respiratory virus, which simply mutates at too great a rate for vaccines to keep up with.

Vaccine Prevents Replication after Infection—F

- Vaccination does not prevent viral replication[20]

One study showed that peak viral loads are similar in vaccinated persons compared with unvaccinated.[21]

Vaccine Prevents Transmission to Others—F

- COVID-19 vaccines do not prevent transmission

In 2021, CDC Director Rochelle Walensky claimed that vaccinated people "do not carry the virus."[22] Shortly thereafter, NIAID Director Anthony Fauci said they would become "dead ends" for the virus.[23]

> "COVID outbreak at CDC gathering infects 181 disease detectives . . . Nearly all of the attendees were vaccinated."
>
> CDC Epidemic Intelligence Service (EIS) Conference April 2023
> Ars Technica 5/30/2023

Neither statement was true, nor was there any evidence at the time in support of those misrepresentations. According to one study in *JAMA Pediatrics*, there is no difference in the rate of transmission between unvaccinated, vaccinated, and boosted children as measured in children infected with COVID-19.[24]

A study in *The Lancet* concluded:

> Fully vaccinated individuals with breakthrough infections have peak viral loads similar to unvaccinated cases and can efficiently transmit infection in household settings, including to fully vaccinated contacts."[25]

Even as early as December 2020, the FDA announced:

> At this time, data are not available to make a determination about how long the vaccine will provide protection, nor is there evidence that the vaccine prevents transmission of SARS-CoV-2 from person to person.[26]

Vaccine Is Approved for Use by the FDA—F

- Vaccines for children under 12 were not approved; they were released under an EUA
- EUA requirements for vaccine safety, effectiveness, and production quality are weak compared with full approval
- Loss of quality control leads to complications and death
- FDA adopts risky authorization strategy
- Vaccines released under EUA do not require informed consent

COVID-19 vaccines available in the US for children under 12 *are not* approved by the FDA. They *are* authorized under an Emergency Use Authorization (EUA).

Many important distinctions exist between what is required to receive EUA authorization compared with full approval via the Biologics License Application

(BLA). These distinctions have a tremendous impact on the potential safety, production quality, and effectiveness of any vaccine.

BLA approval requires thorough clinical trials and extended follow-up of trial participants. EUA approval does not. That's why updated versions of the mRNA COVID-19 vaccines received EUA approval (fall of 2023) for children six months to twelve years old after only minimal animal and human serum testing for antibody responses.[27]

BLA approval also requires more detailed chemistry, manufacturing, and control data (including facility inspections) than EUA. The FDA has indicated that working through the vast amount of data needed for BLA approval takes months . . . which is perfectly aligned with the intensive process that should be followed for vaccine approval, especially where children are concerned.

Variable Batch Quality

Bad things can happen when proper oversight of the vaccine production process is compromised.

For example, in 2021, three lots of Moderna mRNA vaccine totaling more than 1.6 million doses were recalled after thirty-nine vials were found to contain stainless steel shavings due to a manufacturing irregularity.[28] Three people died as a result.

Variability between batches can result in significant differences in vaccine safety and the frequency of serious adverse events. For example, one study found that just 4.2% of the batches accounted for a staggering 71% of adverse events and nearly 50% of all vaccine-related deaths.[29]

FDA Authorization

A Biologics License Application for mRNA was never submitted to nor approved by the FDA for use in children under twelve years. Even worse, the entire EUA process was short-circuited and rushed. There was minimal oversight over the vaccine production process, and there were no randomized, controlled clinical trials to justify COVID-19 vaccine authorization for children. Additionally, the vaccine was never tested in humans for carcinogenesis, mutagenesis, or impact on fertility.

SpikeVAX®, Moderna's mRNA COVID-19 vaccine, is approved for people twelve years and older. However, it was only clinically tested for safety and efficacy on subjects 18 and over, with an average age of 52. Individuals 12-17 years old were tested for neutralizing antibodies but not clinical results.[30]

There has been no testing on children six months to eleven years old, nor has there been FDA approval. Administration of SpikeVAX® to children under twelve is by Emergency Use Authorization.

Comirnaty®, BioNTech and Pfizer's mRNA COVID-19 vaccine, is similarly approved for people twelve and older. Clinical testing for safety and effectiveness for minors included a mix of clinical results and neutralizing antibody testing.

Pfizer's clinical trial results submitted to the FDA on children ages six months to four years serve only to highlight the unreliability of their clinical testing.[31]

Pfizer's clinical trial recruited 4526 children between the ages of six months and four years to receive either three vaccinations or placebo. The groups would then be compared for the relative incidence of COVID-19 infection. Of the initial trial group of 4526 children, 3070 or two-thirds dropped out. The loss of two-thirds of trial participants is extraordinarily high, and casts doubt on the reliability of study methods and results right from the start.[32]

Equally troubling was how COVID-19 infections were excluded from the vaccine group. The interval between the first shot and second was three weeks, and between the second and third shots, eight weeks. One week after the third injection, researchers started counting infections in the vaccinated group. In other words, twelve weeks elapsed between the first shot and the first infections were attributed to the vaccine group. Any cases that occurred during those twelve weeks would be excluded.

For example, in the first three weeks, there were 34 infections in the vaccine group and 13 in the placebo group, but these cases were excluded from calculation of vaccine effectiveness.[33]

After twelve weeks (and 3070 children dropped out of the study), there were 13 cases in the vaccine group and 21 cases in the placebo group, resulting in Pfizer's assertion of vaccine efficacy of 73%. However, the Absolute Risk Reduction was just 3%. And such is the evidence FDA found compelling enough to issue an EUA for Pfizer's mRNA COVID-19 vaccine for children six months to four years of age.[34]

How did the FDA get to this point? During the summer of 2023, the FDA appears to have crossed the line in terms of rationalizing the absence of human clinical trials for vaccine authorization. They recommended authorization of new vaccines based on animal or human antibody responses, not demonstrated clinical safety or effectiveness.[35]

In other words, the FDA bet on a high-risk strategy regarding a completely novel vaccine technology. They based authorization on a theory about how future, unknowable Omicron variants might respond to vaccines based on strains present at the time.

The FDA Knew COVID-19 Vaccine Was Dangerous

At the FDA's Vaccines and Related Biologics Advisory Committee (VRBAC) meeting on October 22, 2022, the committee discussed a working list of serious vaccine adverse events known at the time.[36] This information was not disclosed to the public. Instead, the FDA and CDC repeatedly stated that the vaccine was safe and effective.

The drafted list of possible adverse event outcomes discussed at that meeting included a concerningly long (and serious) list of items:

- Guillain-Barré syndrome
- Acute disseminated encephalomyelitis
- Transverse myelitis
- Encephalitis/myelitis/encephalomyelitis/meningoencephalitis/meningitis/encephalopathy
- Convulsions/seizures
- Stroke
- Narcolepsy and cataplexy
- Anaphylaxis
- Acute myocardial infarction
- Myocarditis/pericarditis
- Autoimmune disease
- Death
- Pregnancy and birth outcomes
- Other acute demyelinating diseases
- Non-anaphylactic allergic reactions
- Thrombocytopenia
- Disseminated intravascular coagulation
- Venous thromboembolism
- Arthritis and arthralgia/joint pain
- Kawasaki disease
- Multisystem Inflammatory Syndrome in Children
- Vaccine enhanced disease

Informed Consent

Children vaccinated for COVID-19 became unknowing test subjects without informed consent.

Why no informed consent? Quite simply, a vaccine or medication that is released under an EUA is exempt from the requirement for informed consent. Remarkably, the Director of Health and Human Services, a non-physician bureaucrat, can declare a public health emergency and approve a request for an EUA.

A simple way to determine if a product has been released under an EUA is to ask for a copy of the package insert required of approved drugs. The inserts disclose all ingredients, clinical trial results, safety information, drug interactions, dosing, etc. Package inserts for vaccines released under an EUA *are blank*. In effect, the FDA, CDC, and manufacturers say, "just trust us."

Keep this in mind as FDA reels off one EUA after another for new COVID-19 and other mRNA vaccines in the pipeline.

The importance of package inserts and how to read them will be discussed in Chapter 21, Five Questions to Ask Your Pediatrician.

Vaccine Safety and Efficacy Supported by Randomized, Controlled, Clinical Trials—F

- Authorized mRNA vaccines were not supported by randomized, controlled clinical trials.
- Reports of vaccine effectiveness were misleading.
- CDC shut down its own COVID-19 safety monitoring system.
- Independent labs, including Canadian government labs, have shown mRNA to be adulterated and that it should be subject to recall.

Are COVID Vaccines Safe & Effective for Children?

In June of 2022, Dr. Ashish Jha (acting head of the White House COVID Task Force at that time), said that data showed the COVID vaccine protects children:

> "Let's set the record straight, because the data here is actually quite clear . . . [k] ids are better protected if they are vaccinated. If they are vaccinated, they are far less likely to get seriously ill. They're far less likely to end up in the hospital, far less likely to end up in the ICU."[37]

But is that what the data says? Actually, there is abundant data that the vaccines are unsafe for children and little evidence for clinical effectiveness. According to Dr. Marty Makary, surgeon and professor at Johns Hopkins University,

> "[T]here has never been a vaccine added to the child immunization schedule without solid clinical evidence that it reduces disease significantly in the community. The COVID vaccine in children will be the first. It will be added with no clinical data."[38]

Newly authorized COVID-19 mRNA vaccines have not been subjected to randomized, controlled, human clinical trials. Information regarding safety and efficacy can only be measured after the fact through post-marketing data collection and analysis.

There have been no published studies on carcinogenesis (causes cancer), mutagenicity (induces genetic mutations), biodistribution (circulation throughout the body), inactivation kinetics (rate of breakdown of synthetic mRNA), or duration of vaccine-induced antigen expression (how long the mRNA keeps producing toxic Spike protein).[39]

In other words, each child is a test subject and there are no placebo controls against which to measure outcomes or safety.

Vaccine Effectiveness

Both Pfizer and Moderna vaccines have been widely reported to be 95% effective at preventing infection–not severe illness, hospitalization, or death–just illness with at least one symptom. This percentage sounds impressive, but few realize it reflects the Relative Risk Reduction (RRR) calculation instead of the Absolute Risk Reduction (ARR).

> Recall from the previous chapter that vaccine manufacturers report effectiveness results via Relative Risk Reduction (RRR). In large vaccine clinical trials, where the disease in question has a low rate of occurrence, the RRR is often skewed toward a positive result. If one wants to know the reduction in risk for a particular child, the Absolute Risk Reduction (ARR) calculation may be more useful, the same one drug manufacturers use when reporting their results.

Vaccine efficacy at preventing illness from COVID-19 for the Pfizer-BioNTech and Moderna mRNA vaccines was reported to be 95%.[40, 41] Of course, the 95% efficacy figure was the RRR calculation. The ARR was only 0.7% for the Pfizer COVID-19 mRNA vaccine and 1.1% for the Moderna COVID-19 vaccine.[42] In other words, COVID-19 vaccination reduced an individual's risk of getting infected by around 1%, not 95%.

An excellent discussion of how RRR was misused in estimating COVID-19 vaccination can be found in this reference.[43]

V-safe System Stops Tracking COVID-19 Vaccines

In 2020, the CDC developed a voluntary monitoring system called "V-safe after vaccination health checker" to specifically monitor the safety of the COVID-19 vaccines.[44] The system was designed to enable patients to report vaccine side effects through the convenience of an online system.

The CDC proudly declared:

> V-safe was developed specifically for COVID-19 vaccines and has been an essential component of the pandemic vaccine safety monitoring systems that have successfully and comprehensively characterized the safety of the COVID-19 vaccines used in the United States.[45]

That is, it *was* an essential component–until the V-safe system revealed a dangerously high 7.7% incidence of severe adverse events (potentially life-threatening), emergency department visits, and hospitalizations.[46]

Apparently, these weren't the results CDC was looking for. They shut down the V-safe program for COVID-19 vaccines in May 2023 and switched the focus of the system to Respiratory Syncytial Virus (RSV).

The V-safe link to COVID-19 vaccines on the CDC site is no longer active.

A Contaminated Vaccine

Drug manufacturers and regulatory agencies have insisted for the past three years that the COVID-19 vaccines were safe. Independent scientists, including Health Canada, however, have now reported Pfizer's mRNA vaccine is contaminated.[47,48,49]

Contaminants consist of DNA plasmids, circular strands of DNA left over from the production process. In a published scientific paper, DNA contamination was reported to be well above allowable limits in vials tested.[50] Unexpected DNA contamination averaged over 100%, resulting in more DNA than mRNA in Pfizer's shot. Moderna's vaccine ran about 50% contamination.[51] In addition, the researchers found up to 186 billion copies of the SV40 cancer promoter gene sequences and virus Spike protein in the DNA contaminant.[52] SV40 poses a risk of altering human DNA, as explained below.

Perhaps most alarming is that contaminated vaccine batches correlated with VAERS serious adverse event reports, suggesting the potential harm of mRNA vaccine contamination is more than theoretical.

The scientists concluded that "these data demonstrate the presence of billions to hundred of billions of DNA molecules per dose in these vaccines" and that "all products tested exceeded the guidelines for residual DNA set by the FDA and WHO by 188 to 509-fold. Our findings extend existing concerns about vaccine safety."[53]

Process 1 and Process 2

The reason for the contamination appears to be that a different manufacturing process was used for vaccine mass production (Process 2) than was used to make vaccines for the clinical trials (Process 1). As will be discussed, Process 2 more readily lends itself to contamination.

The existence of two separate processes was not known until the summer of 2022 when two Israeli researchers noticed that Pfizer amended its clinical trial protocol, making reference to Process 1 and Process 2.[54]

Subsequently, in 2023 a pharmacist was tasked by the court system to review documents a judge forced Pfizer to disclose (documents the company intended to shield from public view for 75 years). The pharmacist found that Pfizer had conducted a smaller trial within their major study. The majority of patients received a vaccine made with Process 1. However, some patients were given vaccines from a different manufacturing process, Process 2, without being informed. The processes turned out to be quite different, with Process 2 showing evidence of considerable contamination.[55]

Manufacturing Process 1 deployed by Pfizer to make the COVID vaccine for the clinical trial used a process akin to a photocopier (polymerase chain reaction, or PCR), making multiple clones of the original mRNA. The PCR process is very precise, but it is expensive and difficult to commercially scale up to produce billions of doses.

Process 2 employs a completely different manufacturing process, one that uses E. coli bacteria to produce mRNA in large batches capable of making millions of doses at a time. Unfortunately, during Process 2, DNA left over from the genetically manipulated E. coli can contaminate the final product, which is what happened in this case. Hence, the DNA plasmid fragments found by the independent researchers noted above, which also happened to contain SV40 genetic material.

The bait and switch should have been disclosed to the public. Moreover, since the FDA knew of the two separate manufacturing processes, they should have required a separate, randomized, controlled clinical trial using vaccine from Process 2 before authorizing its release. Instead, the FDA accepted a secret, limited clinical trial of just a few hundred patients, insufficient to detect a safety signal or to establish effectiveness.

Risk of DNA Contaminants

At least one state surgeon general has called for immediate withdrawal of modRNA COVID-19 vaccines due to the risk of DNA contamination.[56] What is the concern? The FDA itself outlined in a 2007 guidance document the potential for harm, stating there should be certain considerations for vaccines using novel delivery methods, specifically that:

- DNA integration could theoretically impact a human's oncogenes, the genes responsible for transforming a healthy cell into a cancerous cell.
- DNA integration may result in chromosomal instability.
- Biodistribution of DNA vaccines could affect unintended parts of the body including blood, heart, brain, liver, kidney, bone marrow, ovaries/testes, lung, draining lymph nodes, spleen, and the site of administration and subcutis at injection site.[57]

Pfizer itself has said that mRNA technology is a good fit for gene editing, which means of course that the technology can be used to modify human DNA.[58]

Based on their own guidance, it is the FDA's obligation to ensure there is no contaminant DNA integration into the cells of vaccinated persons or evidence of oncogene activation. But the FDA's response to the Florida Surgeon General's inquiry did little to assure the public. A press release from the Surgeon General's Office stated:

> The FDA's response does not provide data or evidence that the DNA integration assessments they recommended themselves have been performed. Instead, they pointed to genotoxicity studies–which are inadequate assessments for DNA integration risk. In addition, they obfuscated the difference between the SV40 promoter/enhancer and SV40 proteins, two elements that are distinct.[59]

FDA Refuses to Recall mRNA Vaccines

Notwithstanding evidence of contamination and calls for the immediate removal of COVID-19 vaccines from the market, the FDA has stated:

> With over a billion doses of the mRNA vaccines administered, no safety concerns related to the sequence of, or amount of, residual DNA have been identified. The FDA stands behind its findings of quality, safety, and efficacy for the mRNA vaccines.[60]

Better evidence of COVID-19 modRNA safety at the molecular level as well as clinical outcomes would help substantiate the FDA's claims. As time goes on, the FDA's assurances of COVID-19 modRNA vaccines' safety and efficacy will likely be judged harshly.

Further details and the implications of the COVID-19 vaccine as a representative model of mRNA vaccines will be taken up in Chapter 17, Why You Should Never, Ever Give a Child an mRNA Vaccine.

Vaccine Does Not Significantly Impact Developing Childhood Immune, Cardiovascular, Neurological, Hematological, Hormonal, or Musculoskeletal Systems—F

- Laboratory-created synthetic Spike proteins are the primary drivers of vaccine injury, whether introduced by mRNA or adenovirus vector vaccines.
- COVID-19 vaccines exert significant, deleterious effects on multiple, immature developing organ systems.
- Adverse events include myocarditis and pericarditis, neurological disorders, infertility, immune suppression, and autoimmune disorders.

Spike Proteins at the Core of Vaccine Injury

Spike proteins are increasingly implicated as the principal cause of vaccine injury.[61] A brief outline of the mechanism by which mRNA-driven Spike protein production leads to organ system damage is provided below.

- The SARS-CoV-2 Spike protein is highly toxic and inflammatory, whether derived from the virus (synthesized in a lab) or created from genetic code in mRNA and adenovector DNA vaccines.
- Lipid nanoparticles that carry the mRNA vaccine genetic code distribute throughout the body within hours after injection into the deltoid muscle, making their way to the brain, heart, reproductive organs, and placenta.
- Unlike mRNA vaccines, viruses (even the lab-created ones) rarely cross the blood-brain barrier or the placenta.

- Lipid nanoparticles are inflammatory themselves and the PEG (polyethylene glycol) component is thought to be a cause of anaphylactic reactions to the vaccine.
- mRNA is actually modified by insertion of a synthetic nucleotide to create a modified RNA or modRNA that helps the modRNA evade immune detection and destruction by enzymes that normally break down mRNA. modRNA may reside in the body for months to years.
- Lab experiments have shown that modRNA may enter the nucleus of cells despite FDA and CDC assurances that this is not possible.
- Production of foreign proteins such as Spike protein on cell surfaces can induce autoimmune responses and tissue damage.
- The Spike protein causes organ system injury through several mechanisms that lead to inflammation, thrombogenesis (creation of blood clots), and damage to the lining of blood vessels.
- Spike protein interaction with tumor suppressor genes may enhance susceptibility to cancer.
- VAERS and FDA-Pfizer reports obtained via FOIA show high rates and multiple organ systems affected, primarily neurological, cardiovascular, and reproductive.
- Repeated COVID-19 vaccine booster doses appear to induce immune system tolerance to SARS-CoV-2 variants and may contribute to recurrent COVID-19 infection and long COVID.

Chapter 17, Why You Should Never, Ever Give a Child an mRNA Vaccine, goes into greater depth on this issue.

Myocarditis

The negative cardiac effects of mRNA vaccines were identified early in the pandemic, so the occurrence of myocarditis following mRNA vaccination should come as no surprise.

The FDA's Office of Vaccines Research and Review warned the manufacturer that their COVID-19 vaccine could result in heart inflammation or myocarditis. As such, they required the manufacturer to include a warning in the package insert about an increased risk of myocarditis and pericarditis following administration of the mRNA vaccine.[62]

The CDC and the American Academy of Pediatrics (AAP) claim that vaccine-induced myocarditis and pericarditis are very rare, and when they do occur, cases are mild. They also posit that heart inflammation from COVID tends to be worse than heart inflammation after vaccination.[63] However, several studies have demonstrated a much higher incidence of myocarditis/pericarditis following vaccination than is acknowledged by the CDC and the American Academy of Pediatrics.[64,65,66] Rates hundreds of times higher than predicted in adolescent boys have been observed.[67]

A peer-reviewed study published in the reputable *European Heart Journal* in early 2024 confirmed that COVID-19 mRNA "booster" shots are dramatically increasing the risk of myocarditis in teenagers and young adults.[68]

The study found that the third dose of Pfizer and Moderna COVID-19 mRNA vaccines was associated with an increased rate of myocarditis of two times and nearly nine times respectively compared to the risk after the second dose.

Heart Damage from Myocarditis

Myocardial injury from myocarditis may only become apparent after months or years and can result in heart failure and death.

For example, one study found the majority of young people who had heart damage from COVID-19 vaccine had residual abnormalities a year later, suggesting a scar could be forming in the heart muscle.[69] Of these, nearly one fifth of cases had evidence of reduced heart function, putting the children at risk for development of heart failure.

Occurrence of Post-Vaccine Myocarditis May Be Much Larger Than Previously Known

About three quarters of young patients in the myocarditis study were initially asymptomatic, with no history of palpitations, chest pain, or shortness of breath. Heart damage was only detected as a result of EKG and lab tests. These findings imply that post-COVID-19 vaccination myocarditis in younger people is being underreported.[70]

Another study of vaccinated thirteen- to eighteen-year-old students found one-fifth had an abnormal EKG post-vaccination. Just as disturbing, 3.5% (all males) had myocarditis or pericarditis, and nearly one-third had cardiovascular effects ranging from tachycardia to palpitations to heart inflammation.[71]

These results stand in stark contrast to a post-COVID-19 infection rate of myocarditis of around 0.002%.[72,73]

Autopsy Study of Vaccine-Induced Myocarditis

A recent review of published autopsy studies of COVID-19 vaccine-induced myocarditis (all ages) suggests there is a high likelihood of a causal link between COVID-19 vaccines and death from suspected myocarditis. This is particularly true in cases of sudden, unexpected death in vaccinated persons.[74]

In terms of risk/benefit of COVID-19 vaccination, the risk of myocarditis in children far outweighs any potential benefit.

Screening of Vaccinated Youths

All young people who have been vaccinated, particularly those who engage in vigorous sports and activities, should undergo a screening EKG and blood tests to detect possible hidden cardiac injury.

Nervous System Toxicity

In a large study of individuals who received at least two doses of COVID-19 vaccines, nearly one-third suffered neurological complications including diplopia (double vision), tremors, muscle spasms, paresthesia (numbness, burning, or prickling sensation), vertigo, brain fog, headaches, sleepiness, taste and smell alterations, and insomnia.[75]

Females were at increased risk of complications. Other risk factors include a history of allergies, immunodeficiency disorders, antitumor medications, transfusions, and previous COVID-19 infection.[76]

Several other studies have reported devastating neurological injuries post COVID-19 vaccination, including cerebral venous thrombosis (a large blood clot in the brain), Guillain-Barré syndrome, transverse myelitis (inflammation of the spinal cord which can lead to paralysis), acute disseminated encephalomyelitis (diffuse, widespread inflammation of the brain), and Bell's palsy.[77,78]

Despite these reports, the American Academy of Neurology and the American Academy of Pediatrics still recommend COVID-19 vaccination for all eligible children under the age of twelve, and as young as six months.[79,80]

Dr. William Makis compiled a list of 33 cases of encephalitis following COVID-19 vaccination in children under 18 extracted from VAERS case reports.[81]

Preliminary Evidence for Autism

Two studies on the COVID-19 vaccine and autism were published in early 2024: one involving lab animals and one involving children exposed in the womb.

In brief, the animal study found that offspring of rats vaccinated during pregnancy had neurodevelopmental disorders similar to autism. These included abnormalities of socialization, motor coordination and balance, quantity of brain Purkinje cells that regulate and coordinate motor movements, and decreased brain-derived proteins that control neuronal development, metabolism, and production of neurotransmitter chemicals.[82]

In the human study published in *JAMA Pediatrics*, researchers compared how well children born to vaccinated mothers met developmental milestones compared with children born to unvaccinated mothers. The authors of the paper concluded that, "in utero exposure to COVID-19 vaccination was not associated with abnormal neurodevelopmental scores on the Ages and Stages Questionnaire, third edition, at 12 or 18 months of life."[83]

However, when boys are looked at separately from girls, a disturbing pattern emerges. At twelve months, there is a statistically significant negative effect on developmental screening tests of maternal COVID-19 vaccination on boys compared with girls. And at eighteen months, there is again a large difference in relative risk between boys versus girls, although it does not achieve statistical significance. The neurodevelopmental effects were most prominent in children of mothers vaccinated during the first trimester compared with the second and third trimesters.[84]

Effect on Fertility

Numerous reports and studies have identified declines in fertility after the introduction of COVID-19 vaccines. These include declining birth rates in multiple countries, increase in spontaneous abortions and stillbirths, and decreased sperm counts after introduction of the vaccines.[85,86,87,88,89,90]

Additionally, the known widespread distribution of mRNA lipid nanoparticles throughout major organ systems, including the ovaries, may pose a risk to girls going through puberty.[91]

mRNA Vaccines May Impair Immune Responses to Non-COVID-19 Infections in Children

Studies before and after a second Pfizer COVID-19 vaccination found a significant decrease in childhood immune response to different types of infections such as bacteria and fungi as well as other viruses.[92] The diminished immune response peaked at one month but persisted for the duration of the study up to six months.

This decreased immunity to other pathogens (acquired immune deficiency) is referred to by some as Vaccine Acquired Immunodeficiency Syndrome (VAIDS).

It remains unclear whether such a phenomenon exists, but outbreaks of potentially deadly staphylococcus and Streptococcus infections in children and adolescents who may have diminished immune response as a contributing factor are concerning. Notably, the rise in infections correlates with vaccinations, not COVID-19 infections.[93,94]

For example, the CDC observed that invasive Strep A infections went down during the COVID-19 pandemic. However, they began to rise in 2022 and stayed high in some parts of the country during 2023.[95]

Immune System Hazard after a Third Dose of mRNA Vaccines

Immunoglobulins, or antibodies, are essential to protect against bacteria, viruses, and fungi. In the case of COVID-19, high levels of neutralizing SARS-CoV-2 antibodies are essential for vaccine-induced immunity. Neutralizing antibodies prevent the virus from entering and infecting cells, keeping them from replicating and causing severe infection.

Shortly after receiving two mRNA vaccine doses, proinflammatory immunoglobulins, specifically IgG1 and IgG3, which are essential for neutralizing invading organisms, increase substantially.

But something remarkable happens after a third dose: anti-COVID-19 antibodies become increasingly composed of non-inflammatory blocking antibodies (IgG4), diminishing the immune response to infections.[96] The switch is so dramatic that the ratio of IgG4 to IgG1&3 increases up to 500-fold after the third vaccination.

This dramatic shift in antibodies blunts the immune response to SARS-CoV-2 and impairs destruction and removal of infectious organisms by immune cells. Persistent elevation of IgG4 can increase cancer susceptibility and predisposition to chronic inflammatory conditions.[97,98]

Autoimmune Disorders

COVID-19 vaccines are known to elicit a powerful immune response, including cytokine storm[99] (when the immune system responds too aggressively to an infection or other immune stimulants like the COVID-19 vaccines). A 2023 study noted, "The short time span between COVID-19 vaccine administration and the onset of R-IMIDs [rheumatic immune-mediated inflammatory diseases] suggests the potential possibility of a cause-and-effect relationship."[100] The hyperactivation of the immune system can lead to life-threatening inflammatory conditions.

New-onset autoimmune disorders after COVID-19 vaccination have also been reported, including immune thrombotic thrombocytopenia, autoimmune liver diseases, Guillain–Barré syndrome, IgA nephropathy, skin disorders, rheumatoid arthritis, and systemic lupus erythematosus.[101,102]

Various theories about the potential causes of COVID-19 vaccine-induced autoimmune disorders exist, but a causal link has not yet been established. However, a number of studies have looked at the association with specific autoimmune disorders. A study led by researchers from the UK's National Health Service examined the cases of people who developed rheumatic diseases after COVID-19 vaccine administration.[103] New onset rheumatic diseases post-vaccination included arthritis, vasculitis, lupus, and adult-onset Still's disease.

Over 80% of these patients developed symptoms after their first or second dose of the COVID-19 vaccine. On average, patients developed rheumatic diseases eleven days after vaccination. Most were treated with steroids. About one-quarter of patients experienced total disease remission, and about 50% improved following treatment. Eight were admitted to intensive care, and two died from their symptoms.

Immune-mediated inflammatory disease describes a cluster of conditions that affect joints, tendons, muscles, blood vessels, and bones and share common inflammatory pathways. Although the exact cause is unknown, advances in molecular research have revealed that an imbalance in inflammatory cytokines is central to their onset.[104]

Vaccine Creates Lifelong Immunity—F

COVID-19 vaccines do not create lifelong immunity. Immunity to circulating variants is short-lived, if at all, and for the multiply vaccinated, there is evidence of negative efficacy (more likely to get the disease compared with fewer or no vaccinations).[105,106,107,108]

Vaccine Essential for Herd Immunity—F

COVID-19 vaccines do not support herd immunity as a consequence of their lack of long-term efficacy.

Overall Grade—F

Healthy children are at low risk of severe illness from COVID-19. Vaccines do not prevent infection, replication, or transmission of the virus. There is evidence of poor controls over the vaccine manufacturing process.

SARS-CoV-2 virus Spike proteins lie at the heart of vaccine injury, affecting virtually every developing organ system. Children's immune systems are harmed from non-sterilizing (don't prevent infection or viral replication) mRNA vaccines, potentially impairing their immune response to new variants and other pathogens.

This discussion about mRNA vaccines continues in Chapter 17, Why You Should Never, Ever Give a Child an mRNA Vaccine.

CHAPTER 5

Hepatitis B—HepB

Hepatitis B (HepB) is FDA approved for children at birth. The rating is attributed in part to the very low incidence of neonates at risk of exposure, ruling out a justification of the recommendation that all newborns be subjected to the risks of HepB vaccination.

Hepatitis B is the most common serious liver infection in the world. It is caused by the hepatitis B virus (HBV) and can result in potentially fatal cirrhosis and liver cancer. Most people who get infected clear the virus naturally, although a small percentage become chronic carriers and can transmit the disease.

Fortunately, HBV is not easy to catch, unlike measles or chickenpox where simple proximity can result in infection. HBV is typically only transmitted through direct contact with infected blood or certain bodily fluids, such as through sharing unsterile needles or contaminated medical equipment or having unprotected sex. The vast majority of infections are sexually transmitted.[1]

Criteria	Grade
Children are at high risk of severe illness or death from disease	F
Vaccine prevents infection and replication	A
Vaccine prevents transmission to others	A
Vaccine is approved for use by the FDA	A
Vaccine safety and efficacy supported by randomized, controlled, clinical trials	D
Vaccine does not significantly impact developing childhood immune, cardiovascular, neurological, hematological, hormonal, or musculoskeletal systems	F
Vaccine creates lifelong immunity	B
Vaccine important to reach herd immunity	D
Overall	**D**

Vaccine Schedule

According to the CDC, the Advisory Committee on Immunization Practices (ACIP) recommends universal hepatitis B vaccination within twenty-four hours of birth, followed by completion of the vaccine series. Children and adolescents nineteen years and older who have not been vaccinated previously should also be vaccinated, per the CDC.

In cases where an infant is born to an HBV-infected woman, the ACIP recommends administration of hepatitis B vaccine and hepatitis B immune globulin (HBIG) within twelve hours of birth, followed by completion of the vaccine series and post-vaccination serologic testing.[2]

The full hepatitis B series typically includes three doses administered within the first twelve to eighteen months of life.[3]

Vaccines Offered

There are two standalone hepatitis B vaccines and two combination vaccines currently available to children in the US.[4]

Standalone

Vaccine	Excipients[5]
Engerix-B®	aluminum hydroxide, yeast protein, sodium chloride, disodium phosphate dihydrate, sodium dihydrogen phosphate dihydrate
Recombivax®	formaldehyde, potassium aluminum sulfate, amorphous aluminum hydroxyphosphate sulfate, yeast protein

Combination

Vaccine	Excipients[6]
Pediarix® (Hep B-DTaP-IPV)	formaldehyde, aluminum hydroxide, aluminum phosphate, sodium chloride, polysorbate 80 (Tween 80), neomycin sulfate, polymyxin B, yeast protein
Vaxelis® (Hep B-DTaP-IPV-Hib)	polysorbate 80, formaldehyde, glutaraldehyde, bovine serum albumin, neomycin, streptomycin sulfate, polymyxin B sulfate, ammonium thiocyanate, yeast protein, aluminum

Contraindications include severe allergic reaction after a previous dose or to a vaccine component and hypersensitivity to yeast.[7]

Children Are at High Risk of Severe Illness or Death from Disease—F

Children are at low risk of severe illness or death from this disease except in very limited circumstances. An infected mother can transmit the virus to their baby during childbirth, although the baby is protected during gestation. A simple blood test can detect HBV infection, and the vast majority of pregnant women are screened during pregnancy.[8]

In the US, chronic carriers who might infect their infants are quite rare, estimated at 0.3% (3 per 1,000 births), although the prevalence of carriers among inner-city minorities can be much higher at 0.4%-1.5%.[9]

Children born to a chronic carrier are at very high risk of contracting the disease and becoming chronic carriers themselves. Therefore, prevention through adequate prenatal testing and HepB immunization is essential in high-risk pregnancies.

Vaccine Prevents Infection and Replication—A

The estimated efficacy of approved vaccines in prevention of chronic hepatitis B in children is around 95%.[10,11] However, it must be noted that the vaccine is only of benefit to children born to HBV-infected or possibly infected mothers or when HBV status is indeterminate at the time of birth.

Vaccine Prevents Transmission to Others—A

The vaccine is highly effective at preventing transmission from an infected mother to child during birth.

Vaccine is Approved for Use by the FDA—A

The vaccine is approved by the FDA.

Vaccine Safety and Efficacy Supported by Randomized, Controlled, Clinical Trials—D

Safety

The FDA was so eager to approve ENGERIX-B® and RECOMBIVAX HB® vaccines that it accepted follow-up data of just five days post-vaccination for infants and four days for children as evidence for safety. For ENGERIX-B®, a total of thirty-six clinical studies were conducted on thousands of healthy adults and children, yet there was no long-term follow up pre-approval. Safety testing was limited to acute reactions, which proved to be a poor predictor of adverse events to follow.

According to the FDA-approved RECOMBIVAX HB® package insert:

> In three clinical studies, 434 doses of RECOMBIVAX HB®, 5 mcg, were administered to 147 healthy infants and children (up to ten years of age) who were monitored for **five days** after each dose (emphasis ours).[12]

According to the FDA-approved ENGERIX-B® package insert:

> In 36 clinical studies, a total of 13,495 doses of ENGERIX-B® were administered to 5,071 healthy adults and children who were initially seronegative for

> hepatitis B markers and healthy neonates. All subjects were monitored for **4 days** post-administration (emphasis mine).[13]

Neither RECOMBIVAX HB® nor ENGERIX-B®, the two HepB vaccines given to infants and children, have been evaluated for their carcinogenic nor mutagenic potential, nor their potential to impair fertility in humans.[14,15]

Limited Control Groups

RECOMBIVAX HB® was compared to itself with one versus two doses or had no control group at all.

ENGERIX-B® was compared to a previous generation product, a plasma-derived vaccine called Heptavax®, and not to a true placebo like saline. As could be expected, adverse reactions limited to the first few days were mostly soreness and fatigue.

Voluntary Reporting of Adverse Events Was High

Post-marketing (post-FDA approval) adverse events tracked via the voluntary VAERS reporting system tell a different story than what emerged from the limited control groups.

During 2005–2015, a total of 20,231 adverse event reports following HepB vaccination among all ages were submitted to VAERS. The majority of primary US reports (78%) were following HepB vaccine administered with other vaccines on the same visit.[16]

Among the 4,444 single-dose HepB-related reports, 6.5% were classified as serious, including 43 deaths; 27 of these were infants less than four weeks old.[17]

Neurological conditions dominate adverse event reports. According to the manufacturer's (pharmaceutical giant GlaxoSmithKline) package insert, which must disclose known complications, reported adverse events include:[18]

- Meningitis
- Encephalitis
- Herpes zoster
- Anaphylaxis
- Hypersensitivity syndrome (a potentially fatal autoimmune disorder)
- Arthritis
- Multiple sclerosis
- Neuropathy
- Guillain-Barré syndrome
- Bell's palsy
- Seizures
- Syncope
- Transverse myelitis (inflammation of the spinal cord that can lead to paralysis)

From the package insert:

> Because these reactions are reported voluntarily from a population of uncertain size, it is not always possible to reliably estimate their frequency or establish a causal relationship to the vaccine.[19]

True enough, but a Harvard vaccine injury study found that fewer than 1% of vaccine adverse events are reported to the VAERS system.[20] The fact that so many catastrophic neurological complications were picked up by a voluntary tracking system raises serious questions about HepB vaccine safety.

Efficacy

According to the manufacturer, protective efficacy was 95% after a three-dose series, beginning within twelve hours of birth, assuming that 70% of unprotected children born to chronically infected mothers would become infected.[21] Up to 90% of infants who become infected through maternal transmission at the time of birth will become chronic carriers.[22]

Vaccine Does Not Significantly Impact Developing Childhood Immune, Cardiovascular, Neurological, Hematological, Hormonal, or Musculoskeletal Systems—F

The extensive list of adverse event reports indicates children are at significant risk of neurological disorders.

Vaccine Creates Lifelong Immunity—B

Immunity after three doses of vaccine during childhood may last thirty years or more, although the actual duration is unknown.[23]

Vaccine Important to Reach Herd Immunity—D

Herd protection from HepB vaccine is only relevant to children of infected mothers. Herd immunity is limited to those at high risk of exposure.

Overall Grade—D

HepB vaccine is extremely effective at preventing perinatal transmission of HepB to the newborn. However, few infants will benefit due to the low prevalence of HBV in pregnant women. There is a high frequency of reported serious adverse events, including a long list of neurological complications.

Withholding the vaccine from at-risk infants would be unethical, therefore a randomized, placebo-controlled trial of children at-risk is not feasible. However, safety monitoring for more than just a few days is certainly warranted. Voluntary reporting of adverse events is insufficient follow-up. At minimum, vaccinated children should be tracked for several years.

Routine HepB vaccination of all children is as much a political decision as it is a public health decision. It is the public health community's effort to appear non-discriminatory against those persons and communities at highest risk.

So all children get the shots–even though only 1 in 333 children is at risk and mothers of the higher risk newborns can be prescreened.

Mothers at low risk who test negative should be informed about the actual risk of infection to their child. They should then be given the option not to vaccinate or delay vaccination of their children unless or until they or their children subsequently fall into a high-risk category or regular caregivers test positive for HepB.

The delay of vaccination in a newborn by a month could have a profound effect on neurodevelopment. Results of a study obtained under a FOIA request to the CDC found that children vaccinated in the first month of life compared with children without vaccination had twofold increased risk for speech delays, fivefold increased risk for sleep disorders, and 7.6-fold increased risk for autism.[24]

If in doubt, vaccinate. But if a mother is low risk and tests negative for HBV, vaccination risks clearly outweigh the benefits. Inclusion of this vaccine on the schedule is largely about equity, not health.

CHAPTER 6

Respiratory Syncytial Virus Monoclonal Antibody (RSV-mAB) Nirsevimab

RSV is a common, highly contagious respiratory virus that causes seasonal lower respiratory tract infections associated with bronchiolitis and pneumonia in infants. Bronchiolitis causes inflammation of the smaller airways in the lungs (called bronchioles), leading to swelling and a buildup of mucus. It's seen most commonly in children under one year of age.

Signs of severe disease include short, shallow, and rapid breathing, flaring of the nostrils, belly breathing, cyanosis (bluish coloring) around the lips, mouth, and fingernails, and poor appetite.

Around 97% of children will have contracted the disease by the time they are two years old. However, infection does not confer immunity as repeat infections can occur during the same RSV season, albeit with milder symptoms.

RSV is the leading cause of hospitalization in infants. An estimated 58,000-80,000 children under five years old are hospitalized due to RSV infection each year (about 4 in 1,000).[1] Hospitalized children who are otherwise healthy have a survival rate of around 99%. Children with suppressed immunity have a much higher mortality rate.[2]

Criteria	**Grade**
Children are at high risk of severe illness or death from disease	**C**
Vaccine prevents infection and replication	**B**
Vaccine prevents transmission to others	**B**
Vaccine is approved for use by the FDA	**NA**
Vaccine safety and efficacy supported by randomized, controlled, clinical trials	**D**
Vaccine does not cause clinically significant alteration of childhood immune, cardiovascular, neurological, hematological, hormonal, or musculoskeletal systems.	**C**

Criteria	Grade
Vaccine creates lifelong immunity	F
Vaccine important to reach herd immunity	F
Overall	**D**

Vaccine Schedule

The CDC recommends that infants younger than eight months who were born during RSV season (fall through spring) receive one dose of nirsevimab if:

- The mother did not receive RSV vaccine during pregnancy.
- The mother's RSV vaccination status is unknown.
- The infant was born within 14 days of maternal RSV vaccination.

Children 8-19 months old who are at increased risk for severe RSV disease and entering their second RSV season should receive an additional dose. This includes:

- American Indian/Alaska Native children.
- Children with chronic lung disease who require medical support during the 6 months before the start of their second RSV season.
- Children who are severely immunocompromised.
- Children with severe cystic fibrosis.

Vaccines Offered

Therapeutic	Excipients[3]
Beyfortus® (nirsevimab)	arginine hydrochloride, histidine, L-histidine hydrochloride monohydrate, polysorbate 80, sucrose

Contraindications include a history of severe allergic reactions to nirsevimab or to any of its components and bleeding disorders. Children who have a moderate or severe acute illness should wait until they recover before getting nirsevimab.

Children Are at High Risk of Severe Illness or Death from Disease—C

Most of the time, RSV causes a mild, cold-like illness. Some cases can progress to severe illness, even in healthy children, although supportive care and pulmonary treatments contribute to high survival rates. In most cases, hospitalization lasts only a few days.[4]

There are an average of 96 RSV deaths per year in children less than one year old (about 2.4 deaths per 100,000).[5] Children with the highest risk for severe illness or death include those born prematurely, those younger than one year old, and those with chronic lung disease, congenital heart disease, weakened immune systems, and neuromuscular disorders.[6]

Vaccine Prevents Infection and Replication—B

During the limited time the monoclonal antibody is effective, it prevents lower respiratory tract infection and replication.

Vaccine Prevents Transmission to Others—B

During the limited time the monoclonal antibody is effective, it prevents transmission to others.

Vaccine Is approved for Use by the FDA—NA

Nirsevimab is a monoclonal antibody therapy, which is an immunoglobulin (immune cell) with anti-RSV activity. It is produced by recombinant DNA technology and works by interfering with RSV's ability to bind to cells and infect them.

Nirsevimab is not a vaccine. It was submitted for approval to the FDA under a Therapeutics Biologic License Application (BLA) as a therapeutic, not a vaccine. As a therapeutic, nirsevimab broke long-standing precedent when added to the vaccine schedule. According to Johns Hopkins Bloomberg School of Public Health,

> Nirsevimab is not a vaccine. It's a preventive drug that offers passive immunity. Monoclonal antibodies work by providing immediate and short-term protection, whereas vaccines boost your immunity in the future.[7]

The addition of nirsevimab to the schedule ensures federal guarantees. The cost of the drug will be covered by the federal Vaccines for Children Program for those that cannot afford it. It also means the manufacturer has blanket protection from liability. No other therapeutic enjoys such a guaranteed income stream or liability protection.

Vaccine Safety and Efficacy Supported by Randomized, Controlled, Clinical Trials—D

Safety

As therapeutics, monoclonal antibodies are intended to treat specific diseases or conditions. For example, monoclonal antibodies have been used to treat COVID-19 as well as certain autoimmune disorders and cancers. However, their use as a preventive therapy for a specific infection like RSV is unprecedented.

The maximum period for follow-up during nirsevimab clinical trials was one year in a limited test group. Long-term effects on millions of children's immunological and other developing systems are simply unknown.

The injection of foreign proteins in the form of monoclonal antibodies into people of any age is known to have significant side effects. According to the Cleveland Clinic,

> Infusion reactions are common after monoclonal antibody treatment. Common signs of infusion reaction are rash, fever, rigor/chills, shortness of breath, changes in blood pressure, and increased heart rate. More serious but less common risks [are] linked to unwanted immune reactions such as anaphylaxis, cytokine release syndrome, and serum sickness.[8]

During nirsevimab's major clinical trial, serious adverse events were 6.8% in the treatment group and 7.3% in the saline placebo group.[9] A higher incidence of adverse events in the control group suggests that the trial was subject to confounding errors in the randomization process. For example, underlying health status and the rate and types of vaccinations received by the respective groups were not reported and may not have been controlled for.

Antidrug antibodies were detected in over 6% of infants who received nirsevimab. This means that the child's immune system attacked the injected antibodies, thereby decreasing their concentration. Two of the twelve infants (16.6%) in the treatment group who had severe respiratory infections had antidrug antibodies.[10]

Carcinogenesis, mutagenesis, and reproductive toxicity studies were not performed.[11]

It should be noted that the clinical trials were paid for by the vaccine manufacturers and developers, AstraZeneca and Sanofi.

Efficacy

The major clinical trial looked at two important outcomes: serious RSV lower respiratory tract infection (LRTI) requiring medical care and hospitalization due to RSV.[12] Relative Risk Reduction for the first outcome was estimated at 74.5% and 62% for hospitalization. The reduction in hospitalization was not statistically significant.

In other words, clinical trials have not shown that nirsevimab reduces hospitalization or mortality.

Moreover, Absolute Risk Reduction for prevention of medically attended RSV LRTI is around 3.75% and for hospitalization is approximately 0.7%, meager to negligible improvements.

As noted, monoclonal antibodies offer passive immunity. They do not stimulate the immune system to develop a lasting immune response as do most vaccines (with the notable exception of COVID-19 mRNA vaccines). The duration of effectiveness of most therapeutic monoclonal antibodies is estimated to be weeks to months, although nirsevimab is said to be of longer duration.[13]

Vaccine Does Not Cause Clinically Significant Alteration of Childhood Immune, Cardiovascular, Neurological, Hematological, Hormonal, or Musculoskeletal Systems—C

It is simply too early to determine the long-term risks of mass administration of nirsevimab to all children.

Vaccine Creates Lifelong Immunity—F

Therapeutic does not contribute to lifelong immunity.

Vaccine Important to Reach Herd Immunity—F

Therapeutic does not contribute to herd immunity.

Overall Grade—D

RSV is a common childhood illness with a low incidence of severe illness and hospitalization for healthy children. For healthy kids who do require hospitalization, supportive care yields high survival rates and limited hospital stays.

Clinical trials show no evidence for reduction in hospitalization or mortality, the very reasons for which mass distribution and use of nirsevimab has been promoted.

Nirsevimab is approved as a therapeutic, not a vaccine. The addition of a therapeutic to the Childhood Immunization Schedule is unprecedented. Clinical trials prior to FDA approval involved relatively small test groups and limited follow up compared with most therapeutics. Placing nirsevimab on the schedule will expose millions of children to the therapy and its risks, the vast majority of whom will suffer little to no ill effects from RSV infection.

Antidrug antibodies were detected in clinical trial participants suggesting that mass administration of a monoclonal antibody therapeutic to healthy children may pose a risk of developing RSV drug resistance in hospitalized babies.

CHAPTER 7

Influenza (Flu) Vaccine

Six million children in the U.S. are affected by the flu every year.[1] According to the CDC, the influenza vaccination reduces flu illnesses, doctor visits, absence from school, and the risk of flu-related hospitalization and death in children.

Symptoms of influenza infection in children typically include fever, headache, muscle pain, dry cough, sore throat, weakness, and fatigue usually lasting less than a week. Children with chronic illness or suppressed immunity are at increased risk of severe illness.

The CDC recommends that *all* children six months and older receive an annual flu shot. Like any vaccine, the influenza vaccination causes the development of antibodies after about two weeks. This vaccine is unique, however, in that its composition changes annually. Each year, the CDC tries to predict which flu strains will be in circulation; manufacturers then design the vaccine accordingly.

As a respiratory virus, influenza mutates rapidly as it travels around the globe presenting an annual challenge to manufacturers to match the vaccine with prevailing strains. As a result, influenza vaccines are marginally effective year after year.[2]

Criteria	**Grade**
Children are at high risk of severe illness or death from disease	**D**
Vaccine prevents infection and replication	**D**
Vaccine prevents transmission to others	**D**
Vaccine is approved for use by the FDA	**A**
Vaccine safety and efficacy supported by randomized, controlled, clinical trials	**D**
Vaccine does not significantly impact developing childhood immune, cardiovascular, neurological, hematological, hormonal, or musculoskeletal systems	**D**
Vaccine creates lifelong immunity	**F**
Vaccine important to reach herd immunity	**F**
Overall Grade	**D**

Vaccine Schedule

The CDC recommends that anyone six months of age and older receive the influenza vaccination. Some children require two doses (administered at least four months apart.)[3]

Vaccines Offered

There are two influenza vaccine options, as per the CDC:[4]

1. Flu shots: Given as an injection (with a needle) and approved for use in people six months and older. Indications vary by vaccine.
2. Nasal spray vaccine (LAIV4 = Live Attenuated Influenza Vaccine): Approved for use in non-pregnant, healthy people ages two to forty-nine. Contraindications include asthma, weakened immune systems, taking aspirin or salicylate-containing medications, kidney disease, and the presence of neuromuscular disorders.

There are three general categories of influenza vaccines used for children:[5]

1. Quadrivalent Flu Vaccines: Protect against four different flu viruses.
2. Cell-based Flu Vaccines (Flucelvax Quadrivalent): Grown in mammal cell culture instead of in hens' eggs. This vaccine is completely egg-free and is approved for people six months and older.
3. Nasal Spray Flu Vaccine (Live Attenuated Influenza Vaccine, LAIV4, FluMist Quadrivalent): Given as a nasal spray. This vaccine is made with attenuated (weakened) live flu viruses. It is approved for use in people ages two to forty-nine years. This vaccine is not recommended for use in pregnant women, immunocompromised people, or those with certain medical conditions.

Within these categories, there are several vaccine options:

Age	Category	Manufacturer	Excipients[6]
6+ months (higher dosage given to 3+ years)	Afluria Quadrivalent	Seqirus	sodium chloride, monobasic sodium phosphate, dibasic sodium phosphate, monobasic potassium phosphate, potassium chloride, calcium chloride, sodium taurodeoxycholate, ovalbumin, sucrose, neomycin sulfate, polymyxin B, betapropiolactone, hydrocortisone, thimerosal (multi-dose vials)

Age	Category	Manufacturer	Excipients
6+ months	Fluarix Quadrivalent	GaxoSmithKline	octoxynol-10 (TRITON X-100), α-tocopheryl hydrogen succinate, polysorbate 80 (Tween 80), hydrocortisone, gentamicin sulfate, ovalbumin, formaldehyde, sodium deoxycholate, sodium phosphate-buffered isotonic sodium chloride
6+ months	FluLaval Quadrivalent	GaxoSmithKline	ovalbumin, formaldehyde, sodium deoxycholate, α-tocopheryl hydrogen succinate, polysorbate 80, phosphate-buffered saline solution
6+ months	Fluzone Quadrivalent	Sanofi Pasteur	formaldehyde, egg protein, octylphenol ethoxylate (Triton X-100), sodium phosphate-buffered isotonic sodium chloride solution, thimerosal (multi-dose vials)
6+ months	Flucelvax Quadrivalent	Seqirus	Madin Darby Canine Kidney (MDCK) cell protein, phosphate buffered saline, protein other than HA, MDCK cell DNA, polysorbate 80, cetyltrimethlyammonium bromide, and β-propiolactone, thimerosal (multi-dose vials)
2–49 years	FluMist Quadrivalent	AstraZeneca	monosodium glutamate, hydrolyzed porcine gelatin, arginine, sucrose, dibasic potassium phosphate, monobasic potassium phosphate, ovalbumin, gentamicin sulfate, ethylenediaminetetraacetic acid (EDTA)

Table 2: Influenza vaccine: United States, 2023–24 influenza season[7]

Children Are at High Risk of Severe Illness or Death from Disease—D

Children are not at high risk of severe illness or death from influenza.

The CDC reports the following statistics concerning the flu:

- Children younger than five, and especially those younger than two, have an increased risk of developing serious flu-related complications.[8]
- Children of any age with certain chronic health conditions are also at higher risk: 66% of children (0-17 years old) hospitalized with the flu had at least one underlying health condition. These included asthma,[9] neurologic disease,[10] obesity, and immune suppression. More information is available concerning children at higher risk[11] of potentially serious flu complications.

Among reported pediatric flu deaths:[12]

- 44% of deaths occurred in children younger than five years
  - 14% of these occurred in children younger than six months, and thus too young for the flu vaccine
- 56% of deaths occurred in children ages 5-17 years
- Of the 183 pediatric deaths (among children with medical history on record), 78 (43%) had a pre-existing medical condition[13]

Vaccine Prevents Infection and Replication—D

Influenza vaccines provide inconsistent protection against infection and replication. See the section on Vaccine Safety and Efficacy below.

Vaccine Prevents Transmission to Others—D

Influenza vaccines provide inconsistent protection against transmission. See the section on Vaccine Safety and Efficacy below.

Vaccine is Approved for Use by the FDA—A

Vaccines are approved for use by the FDA.

Vaccine Safety and Efficacy Supported by Randomized, Controlled, Clinical Trials—D

Safety

Post-marketing studies of influenza vaccines (which they are required to do after a vaccine is approved and marketed) have identified Serious Adverse Events reported by manufacturers in the vaccine package insert. Here is a partial list:[14]

- Blood and Lymphatic System Disorders: Thrombocytopenia (decrease in platelets needed for blood coagulation)

- Immune System Disorders: Anaphylaxis, other allergic/hypersensitivity reactions (including urticaria and angioedema)
- Nervous System Disorders: Guillain-Barré syndrome (GBS), convulsions, febrile convulsions, myelitis (including encephalomyelitis and transverse myelitis), facial palsy (Bell's palsy), optic neuritis/neuropathy, brachial neuritis, syncope, dizziness, and paresthesia
- Vascular Disorders: Vasculitis (inflammation of the arteries)
- Respiratory: Dyspnea, cough, wheezing
- Skin and Subcutaneous Tissue Disorders: Rash, pruritus, and Stevens-Johnson syndrome (a potentially deadly immune system reaction where the skin blisters and sloughs off like third-degree burns)

Common adverse events and solicited adverse events, where a manufacturer actively looks for post-vaccination complications, includes the following for children 6-35 months old:[15]

- In children 6-35 months of age, the most common (≥10%) injection-site reactions were pain (57%) or tenderness (47%- 54%), erythema (23%-37%), and swelling (13%-22%); the most common solicited systemic adverse reactions were irritability (47%- 54%), abnormal crying (33%-41%), malaise (38%), drowsiness (31%- 38%), appetite loss (27%-32%), myalgia (27%), vomiting (10%-15%), and fever (11%-14%). (6.1)
- In children 3-8 years of age, the most common (≥10%) injection-site reactions were pain (67%), erythema (34%), and swelling (25%); the most common solicited systemic adverse reactions were myalgia (39%), malaise (32%), and headache (23%). (6.1)

Clearly, the high frequency of systemic adverse events, especially in the 6-35 months group, is a risk that outweighs the modest benefits of vaccination. The 3–8 year-old group doesn't fare much better with an extensive list of systemic adverse events.

Consistent with other childhood vaccines, flu vaccines have not been evaluated for carcinogenic or mutagenic potential, or for impairment of male fertility in animals.[16]

Does Childhood Vaccination Put the Elderly at Increased Risk of Influenza?

Cambridge University Press published a study that found repeated vaccination at a young age may double the risk of influenza in older populations "solely due to differences between vaccine-induced immunity and naturally acquired immunity."

(Continued on next page)

The study also suggests that the "possible benefits of [continuously] vaccinating otherwise healthy children over 5 years of age . . . could be outweighed by severe clinical consequences and increased costs in the elderly." A notable take-away from this article is the statement, "unlike vaccination, naturally acquired immunity can provide long-lasting protection against subsequent infection by the same viral subtype."[17]

Effectiveness

In 2018, the Cochrane Library published an important review of forty-one clinical trials of influenza vaccine with over 200,000 child participants, most of whom were two-plus years old.[18] Cochrane reviews are considered the gold standard for meta-analysis (retrospective analysis of previous scientific publications where data is pooled across several studies and the results are reanalyzed).The trials compared live attenuated and inactivated vaccines with placebo or no vaccine, and the resulting numbers support the re-evaluation of the push to administer influenza vaccine to all children.

Here are the details:

Live attenuated vaccines

Compared with placebo/no vaccine, the Cochrane Study found that live attenuated influenza vaccines likely reduce the risk of influenza infection in children 3-16 years old from 18% to 4%, and they may reduce influenza-like illness (ILI) by a smaller degree, from 17% to 12%.

Influenza-like illness (ILI) is defined as the presence of fever of greater than or equal to 100°F, in addition to cough or sore throat, in the absence of an alternative cause. Causes of ILI include respiratory syncytial virus, rhinovirus, adenovirus, parainfluenza viruses, and human coronaviruses.

In other words, seven children (2+ years old) would need to be vaccinated to prevent a single case of influenza, and twenty children would need to be vaccinated to prevent one child from experiencing an ILI.

Inactivated Vaccines (Injected)

Compared with placebo or no vaccination, inactivated vaccines may reduce the risk of influenza in children ages 2-16 years from 30% to 11%, and they probably reduce ILI from 28% to 20%.

Five children would need to be vaccinated to prevent one case of influenza, and twelve children would need to be vaccinated to avoid one case of ILI.

Considering 50% efficacy is considered an important threshold for vaccine approval, the low risk reduction results in the Cochrane Study fail to justify the benefits versus the risks for influenza vaccination of children.

Increased Risk?

Influenza vaccines may actually *increase* children's risk of hospitalization. One study of 261 children (6 months–18 years) found that "infected children were 267% more likely to be hospitalized if they had previously received an influenza [trivalent inactivated] vaccine."[19]

In another randomized study, 69 children received trivalent inactivated influenza vaccination, and 46 received a placebo. Of those vaccinated, 29% developed an infection with a non-influenza upper respiratory virus, whereas 3.4% of those who were not vaccinated developed an upper respiratory infection from a non-influenza virus.[20]

The numbers are small, but a picture of limited benefits is emerging.

Benefits Overstated

Unfortunately, the CDC has had a tendency to overstate the benefits of influenza vaccination. A 2013 article published in the *Journal of the American Medical Association* presented strong evidence that health authorities consistently exaggerate the dangers of the flu and inflate the benefits of influenza vaccination[21] (years later, the same author also correctly identified numerous red flags in the COVID vaccine trials[22]).

A separate article published the same year in the *British Medical Journal* claimed that marketing strategies designed to increase influenza vaccinations lacked moral integrity and scientific support.[23]

Vaccine Does Not Significantly Impact Developing Childhood Immune, Cardiovascular, Neurological, Hematological, Hormonal, or Musculoskeletal Systems—D

Post-marketing and solicited adverse events studies noted above indicated a significant risk of potential injury to various childhood systems in development.

Vaccine Creates Lifelong Immunity—F

Vaccination does not result in lifelong immunity.

Herd Immunity—F

Regular influenza vaccination does not lead to herd immunity. A Cochrane Review did not find evidence that vaccinating children against influenza had any impact on community transmission.[24] This means getting the flu shot to "protect grandma" is a marketing strategy and not grounded in reality.

Notably, "trivalent inactivated vaccination has few effects and there is no evidence that it affects deaths, complications, or transmission of influenza. Live attenuated vaccination performed a little better at the expense of safety."[25]

Overall—D

There is considerable evidence that influenza vaccine effectiveness is low and may even make infection more likely. There is no evidence of community protection resulting from childhood immunization, a common argument for the flu shot. The final determinant of this vaccine's poor overall grade is that systemic adverse events are common, especially in those under three years old.

CHAPTER 8

Diphtheria, Tetanus, acellular Pertussis—DTaP

DTaP vaccine is intended to prevent illness from diphtheria, tetanus, and pertussis. Diphtheria and pertussis spread from person to person. Tetanus enters the body through cuts or wounds. DTaP is a combination vaccine, and each component presents a distinct risk-to-benefit profile.

Development of combination vaccines to protect against multiple diseases began with the combining of diphtheria, tetanus, and pertussis (DTP) vaccines in 1948.[1] DTP was discontinued in favor of DTaP in 1997 due to the high incidence of adverse events using the whole cell pertussis vaccine.

DTaP covers three diseases of bacterial origin, but two of the vaccines, diphtheria and tetanus, don't prevent infection. Instead, they interfere with exotoxins produced by the bacteria after infection has occurred (exotoxins are proteins secreted by the bacteria that can damage the body's cells). Both the diphtheria and tetanus components of the vaccine contain inactivated forms of the exotoxin that trigger the body to create antibodies to the toxins to block their effect.

	Diph	**Tet**	**aP**
Criteria	**Grade**	**Grade**	**Grade**
Children are at high risk of severe illness or death from disease	**D**	**B**	**B**
Vaccine prevents infection and replication	**NA**	**NA**	**C**
Vaccine prevents transmission to others	**NA**	**NA**	**C**
Vaccine is approved for use by the FDA	**A**	**A**	**A**
Vaccine safety and efficacy supported by randomized, controlled, clinical trials	**C**	**C**	**C**
Vaccine does not significantly impact developing childhood immune, cardiovascular, neurological, hematological, hormonal, or musculoskeletal systems	**D**	**C**	**D**

(Continued on next page)

Criteria	Diph Grade	Tet Grade	aP Grade
Vaccine creates lifelong immunity	D	D	D
Vaccine important to reach herd immunity	D	NA	D
Overall Grade	D	B	C

Vaccine Schedule

The CDC states all children should receive six doses of the DTaP vaccine over the first twelve years of life. Infants need three shots of DTaP to build protection. Two additional booster shots are recommended during early childhood, along with an additional shot in the pre-teen years.

DTaP is administered on the following schedule:

- 2 months
- 4 months
- 6 months
- 15-18 months
- 4-6 years
- 11-12 years

Children who cannot or should not receive the DTaP vaccine can be given Td (for tetanus and diphtheria only), but it is unlikely to provide the same levels of protection against diphtheria as DTaP and provides no protection against whooping cough.[2]

DTaP Vaccines Offered

Currently, there are seven pediatric DTaP vaccines licensed in the United States. Two are standalone and five are part of combination vaccines:[3]
Standalone

Vaccine	Excipients[4]
Daptacel®	aluminum phosphate, formaldehyde, glutaraldehyde, 2-phenoxyethanol
Infanrix®	formaldehyde, aluminum hydroxide, sodium chloride, polysorbate 80 (Tween 80)

Combination

Vaccine	Excipients[5]
Kinrix® (DTaP-IPV)	formaldehyde, aluminum hydroxide, sodium chloride, polysorbate 80 (Tween 80), neomycin sulfate, polymyxin B

Vaccine	Excipients
Pediarix® (DTaP-HepB-IPV)	formaldehyde, aluminum hydroxide, aluminum phosphate, sodium chloride, polysorbate 80 (Tween 80), neomycin sulfate, polymyxin B, yeast protein
Pentacel® (DTaP-IPV/Hib)	aluminum phosphate, polysorbate 80, sucrose, formaldehyde, glutaraldehyde, bovine serum albumin, 2-phenoxyethanol, neomycin, polymyxin B sulfate
Quadracel® (DTaP-IPV)	formaldehyde, aluminum phosphate, 2-phenoxyethanol, polysorbate 80, glutaraldehyde, neomycin, polymyxin B sulfate, bovine serum albumin
Vaxelis® (DTaP-IPV-Hib-HepB)	polysorbate 80, formaldehyde, glutaraldehyde, bovine serum albumin, neomycin, streptomycin sulfate, polymyxin B sulfate, ammonium thiocyanate, yeast protein, aluminum

Contraindications include severe allergic reaction after a previous dose, or to a vaccine component, and encephalopathy that is not attributable to another identifiable cause within seven days of administration of a dose of DTP or DT.

DTaP vs Tdap Booster

DTaP is the vaccine for infants and children under seven. Children over seven and adults receive the Tdap vaccine, which has a reduced dose of the diphtheria and pertussis vaccines. The CDC refers to Tdap as a "booster dose" because it boosts the immunity that wanes from earlier DTaP doses.

Diphtheria

Criteria	Grade
Children are at high risk of severe illness or death from disease	**D**
Vaccine prevents infection and replication	**NA**
Vaccine prevents transmission to others	**NA**
Vaccine is approved for use by the FDA	**A**
Vaccine safety and efficacy supported by randomized, controlled, clinical trials	**C**
Vaccine does not significantly impact developing childhood immune, cardiovascular, neurological, hematological, hormonal, or musculoskeletal systems	**D**
Vaccine creates lifelong immunity	**D**
Vaccine important to reach herd immunity	**D**
Diphtheria Vaccine Overall Grade	**D**

The main sites of diphtheria infection are the mucous membranes of the nasopharynx and tonsils and the skin. When the throat and nasal passages are affected, swallowing becomes difficult and there is an increased risk of choking. Diphtheria exotoxin can travel from sites of infection to remote organs including the heart, nervous system, and kidneys.

The disease spreads primarily through droplets, but infection can also result from skin contact.

Children Are at High Risk of Severe Illness or Death from Disease—D

Children are not at high risk of severe illness or death. Diphtheria is extremely rare in the US, and there are excellent treatments for the disease when it is diagnosed early. These include antibiotics to treat the infection and antitoxin serum to block the exotoxin in addition to supportive care.

The Vaccine Does Not Prevent Infection, Replication, or Transmission—NA

The vaccine works only by blocking the effect of the exotoxin. It has no effect on bacterial infection, replication, or transmission.

The Vaccine is Approved for Use by the FDA—A

The vaccine is approved by the FDA.

Vaccine Safety and Efficacy Supported by Randomized, Controlled, Clinical Trials—C

Safety

Safety clinical studies on DTaP vaccine have only been conducted against DTP, DT, or other vaccines (Hib, IPV, PCV) as controls. Both groups have high rates of systemic side effects post-vaccination, therefore the manufacturers can claim there were no safety issues compared with "placebos."

Systemic effects for both commercial DTaP vaccines were similar, including: fussiness/irritability (32-75%); anorexia (11-25%); drowsiness (32-36%%); lethargy (51%); and inconsolable crying (58%).[6,7]

Post-marketing surveillance across both commercial DTaP vaccines identified several severe adverse events, the rates of which are unknown due to the random nature of their reporting. They include:

- Bronchitis
- Cough
- Skin infection
- Swollen lymph glands
- Low platelet count
- Encephalopathy
- Cyanosis (bluish color of skin, nail beds, or lips due to low oxygen levels)

- Nausea
- Diarrhea
- Allergic reaction
- Anaphylactic reaction
- Skin rashes
- Seizures
- Loss of consciousness
- Screaming
- SIDS

According to the CDC, DTaP and Tdap vaccines are safe and effective at preventing diphtheria, tetanus, and pertussis.[8] They cite a 2018 study published in *Pediatrics* as evidence for DTaP safety,[9] along with their own review of over 50,000 DTaP adverse events reported to the VAERS database between 1991 and 2016. However, a closer look at the data reveals that over 11% of adverse events were considered serious, and of the serious adverse events (SAE), 15% were deaths.[10]

Depending on the vaccine being studied, an SAE is typically defined as an adverse event that results in any of the following conditions: death; life-threatening at the time of the event; inpatient hospitalization or prolongation of existing hospitalization; emergency department visit; persistent or significant disability/incapacity; a congenital anomaly/birth defect; or a medically important event, based on medical judgment.[11]

It is important to note that VAERS is a voluntary reporting system whose forms require a significant amount of time for health-care professionals to complete. Misrepresentation of facts also carries significant penalties. So it should come as no surprise that busy clinicians often fail to submit the reports. In fact, Harvard researchers estimate that clinicians report as few as 1% of significant adverse events.[12] Were this underreporting estimate to hold for DTaP vaccination, actual SAEs exceeded a half million, including 80,000 deaths over a fifteen-year period.

The VAERS analysis revealed other serious but non-fatal SAEs including fever, vomiting, febrile seizures, diarrhea, and muscle weakness.[13]

Excipients

Both TDaP brands contain aluminum salts, plus other ingredients such as formaldehyde, glutaraldehyde, and polysorbate 80. Aluminum is a powerful adjuvant and the remainder are known toxins. Aluminum toxicity is discussed in greater detail in Chapter 2, First, Do No Harm.

DTaP and SIDS

Almost half of deaths reported to VAERS following DTaP vaccination were reported as sudden infant death syndrome (SIDS) and nearly always in children under six months of age.

Although the CDC is quick to dismiss a causal link between childhood vaccines and SIDS, the fact that SIDS most commonly occurs between ages two to four months, the same brief interval where babies receive twelve vaccines, is an obvious cause for concern.

DTaP and Autism

Upwards of 40% of parents believe that vaccines cause autism.[14] The only study that examined DTaP and autism did find a correlation, albeit based on VAERS reports; the vaccine, at the time, contained Thimerosal.[15] Thimerosal has since been removed from DTaP vaccines due to concerns about neurotoxicity. The excipient has been replaced with either aluminum hydroxide or aluminum phosphate, both also known to have nervous system toxicity.

Subsequently, the Department of Health and Human Services requested the Institute of Medicine (IOM) investigate the issue of vaccines and autism, and DTaP and autism in particular. Despite the CDC's unequivocal assertion that vaccines do not cause autism, the IOM was forced to concede that they just don't know:

Causality Conclusion: The evidence is inadequate to accept or reject a causal relationship between diphtheria toxoid-, tetanus toxoid-, or acellular pertussis-containing vaccine and autism.[16]

Efficacy

Efficacy studies for DTaP have only looked at diphtheria antitoxin levels and not clinical outcomes. This means that vaccinated children were tested for the presence of antitoxins that are generated by the immune system in response to the vaccine but not for whether diphtheria infection was prevented. 98.5% of those children tested after three doses exceeded a threshold felt to represent necessary levels for protection from infection.

The CDC acknowledges:

> No one has ever studied the efficacy of tetanus toxoid and diphtheria toxoid in a vaccine trial. However, experts infer efficacy from protective antitoxin levels.[17]

Vaccine Does Not Significantly Impact Developing Childhood Immune, Cardiovascular, Neurological, Hematological, Hormonal, or Musculoskeletal Systems—D

The presence of aluminum in both commercial versions of DTaP vaccine along with the post-marketing adverse event reports suggest the vaccine poses a risk to developing immune, nervous, hematologic, and cardiovascular systems. See below for a discussion of potential harms including Autism and SIDS.

Vaccine Creates Lifelong Immunity—D

There is no evidence for lifelong immunity.

Vaccine Important to Reach Herd Immunity—D

Widespread DTaP vaccination does not contribute to herd immunity.

Overall Grade—D

The benefits do not outweigh the risks in healthy children. Diphtheria is rare in the US and excellent treatments are available. The vaccine exposes children to aluminum salts and other toxic excipients.

Immunocompromised children should be considered high risk for any of these diseases and may derive greater benefit compared with risks than healthy children.

Tetanus

Criteria	Grade
Children are at high risk of severe illness or death from disease	**B**
Vaccine prevents infection and replication	**NA**
Vaccine prevents transmission to others	**NA**
Vaccine is approved for use by the FDA	**A**
Vaccine safety and efficacy supported by randomized, controlled, clinical trials	**C**
Vaccine does not significantly impact developing childhood immune, cardiovascular, neurological, hematological, hormonal, or musculoskeletal systems	**C**
Vaccine creates lifelong immunity	**D**
Vaccine important to reach herd immunity	**NA**
Tetanus Vaccine Overall Grade	**B**

As with diphtheria, tetanus infections produce an exotoxin. Tetanus exotoxin is highly dangerous and spreads throughout the body, interfering with nerve signals to the muscles. The result is sustained muscle contractions, notably in the jaw which causes an unbreakable (and painful) clenching referred to as lockjaw.

Tetanus is not spread between people. It is contracted when bacterial spores found in the soil contaminate a wound that deeply penetrates the skin. Deep in the subcutaneous tissue, tetanus spores germinate and produce a toxin that enters the bloodstream. Once muscle spasm has set in, mortality is quite high.

Wearing proper footwear and vigorously irrigating and cleaning deep wounds are the best preventive measures. Tetanus immune globulin may be used to treat highly contaminated wounds in individuals who are partially vaccinated or unvaccinated.[18] Previous infection does not confer immunity, and fewer than thirty cases per year are recorded in the US.

Children Are at High Risk of Severe Illness or Death from Disease—B

Children are not at high risk and excellent treatments are available if high risk, penetrating wounds are promptly treated.

Vaccine Prevents Infection and Replication or Transmission to Others—NA

Tetanus is caused by an exotoxin, not a bacterial disease. The vaccine does not prevent infection, replication, or transmission of an exotoxin.

Vaccine is Approved for Use by the FDA—A

The vaccine is approved by the FDA.

Vaccine Safety and Efficacy Supported by Randomized, Controlled, Clinical Trials—C

Please refer to the discussion of vaccine safety above. As a combination vaccine, it is not possible to distinguish the safety effects of the tetanus vaccine antigens from the diphtheria and pertussis antigens. The inability to distinguish safety signals related to any one antigen represents a major concern about combination vaccines.

Efficacy studies for DTaP have only looked at tetanus antitoxin levels and not clinical outcomes. This means that vaccinated children were tested for the presence of antitoxins that are generated by the immune system in response to the vaccine but not for whether clinical tetanus was prevented. One hundred percent of those children tested after three doses exceeded a threshold felt to represent necessary levels for protection from infection.

As noted above regarding diphtheria antitoxin levels, the CDC acknowledges,

> No one has ever studied the efficacy of tetanus toxoid and diphtheria toxoid in a vaccine trial. However, experts infer efficacy from protective antitoxin levels.[19]

Vaccine Does Not Significantly Impact Developing Childhood Immune, Cardiovascular, Neurological, Hematological, Hormonal, or Musculoskeletal Systems—C

The lack of placebo comparisons, the presence of aluminum compound excipients, and significant reports of adverse events suggest developing organ systems may be at risk of significant impact.

Vaccine Creates Lifelong Immunity—D

There is no evidence for lifelong immunity. Current recommendations are for a booster shot every ten years, except for a wound that is dirty or tetanus-prone, then a booster is recommended if the last tetanus shot was greater than five years ago.

Vaccine Important to Create Herd Immunity—NA

The vaccine blocks the effect of the exotoxin and has no effect on transmission to others.

Tetanus Overall Grade—B

The benefits may outweigh the risks when it comes to being vaccinated for tetanus, especially given the treatments available. The best prevention is thorough cleansing and debridement of deep wounds. A tetanus booster may be given post-exposure within forty-eight hours of injury, and in cases where a person is high risk or unvaccinated, tetanus immune globulin can be considered.[20] Finally, DTaP exposes children to aluminum salts and other toxic excipients.

Pertussis

Criteria	Grade
Children are at high risk of severe illness or death from disease	**B**
Vaccine prevents infection and replication	**C**
Vaccine prevents transmission to others	**C**
Vaccine is approved for use by the FDA	**A**
Vaccine safety and efficacy supported by randomized, controlled, clinical trials	**C**
Vaccine does not significantly impact developing childhood immune, cardiovascular, neurological, hematological, hormonal, or musculoskeletal systems	**D**
Vaccine creates lifelong immunity	**D**
Vaccine important to reach herd immunity	**D**
Pertussis Vaccine Overall Grade	**C**

Pertussis, also known as whooping cough, can cause severe respiratory symptoms characterized by uncontrollable, violent coughing that makes it difficult to breathe.

Infants and young children are particularly vulnerable as infection can cause pneumonia, seizures, and brain injury.

When indicated, early treatment with antibiotics is highly effective. Most cases resolve without antibiotics after two to three weeks. In one study of severe cases that required hospitalization, 90% were infants.[21] Notably, the inpatient case fatality rate for children is less than 1%.

According to the CDC, there has been an increasing trend in reported cases since the 1980s, despite widespread vaccination.[22] Among the potential causes behind the rising trend, the CDC notes increased awareness, better reporting, and waning immunity. Waning immunity is most likely the consequence of a significant change in vaccine composition in the early nineties.

In 1991, the CDC's Advisory Committee on Immunization Practices (ACIP) recommended modification of the original whole-cell pertussis vaccine due to the high incidence of adverse events. These included seizures, Guillain-Barré Syndrome, encephalitis, coma, and death.

Over the course of six years, manufacturers introduced an acellular (absent cell components) vaccine, DTaP, which completely replaced the whole-cell version by 1997.

However, the trade-off in safety resulted in a less effective vaccine.[23] For example, only 71% of young children have immunity to infection 5 years after getting their fifth dose of DTaP.[24] The results are worse in adolescents, where only 34% have immunity just 2 to 4 years after vaccination.[25]

Children Are at High Risk of Severe Illness or Death from Disease—B

Children are most vulnerable to severe illness during the three months prior to receiving the vaccine. This serves as the basis for the CDC's recommendation that pregnant women receive the Tdap (not DTaP) vaccine to pass along maternal antibodies to the fetus. However, the manufacturer notes,

> A study of immune responses of infants born to mothers who received Tdap during pregnancy found diminished antibody responses to pertussis antigens compared with infants whose mothers received placebo during pregnancy.[26]

Moreover, a diminished *immune response* has been observed in vaccinated infants born to mothers who received Tdap during pregnancy compared with infants born to unvaccinated mothers.[27] The clinical implications of this are not known.

In the author's experience, severe and even deadly pertussis infection in young children is often cited by pediatricians and other providers as justification for DTaP vaccine. Without question, such tragic cases leave a lasting impression on families and providers alike. It is not clear how many of these children were premature or had other pre-existing conditions which may have predisposed them to a poor outcome. Therefore, the risk-benefit calculation may favor use of DTaP in high-risk children.

However, as noted above in the diphtheria discussion on vaccine safety, DTaP vaccination has a high rate of severe adverse events (SAE), and a 15% death rate for children who have a SAE. The number of severe adverse events or deaths caused by the vaccine in order to prevent one pertussis death is not known. It is essential for providers to consider and balance the high rate of vaccine complications with the understandable concern for the rare disability or death resulting from pertussis infection in healthy children.

Fortunately, the vast majority of healthy children who contract pertussis do not develop severe illness or require hospitalization. As noted, the mortality rate for the sickest of infants who require hospitalization is less than 1%. Early antibiotic therapy and supportive care are highly effective treatments.

Vaccine Prevents Infection, Replication, or Transmission to Others—C

Over the past thirty years, pertussis has resurged in the US. Introduction of the acellular vaccine accelerated this phenomenon.[28]

Observational studies concluded that children vaccinated with the acellular vaccines had a two-to-five-fold greater risk of pertussis diagnosis compared with the whole cell version.[29,30] Researchers from the FDA's Center for Biologics Evaluation and Research (CBER) have shown that animals vaccinated with the whole cell vaccine clear infection twice as fast as those vaccinated with the acellular version.[31]

Notably, neither vaccine prevented colonization (infection), and vaccinated primates transmitted the virus to unvaccinated cage mates.[32]

Observational studies of household contacts have shown that asymptomatic pertussis can occur in vaccinated children and adults.[33] Consequently, the FDA's CBER researchers theorized that the pertussis resurgence may be due to acellular vaccinated individuals serving as asymptomatic or mildly symptomatic carriers, thereby contributing significantly to transmission in the population.[34]

Authors of the FDA study conclude,

> Together these data form the key finding of this study: aP [acellular] vaccines do not prevent infection or transmission of *Bordetella pertussis* even 1 month after completing the primary vaccination series.[35]

Vaccine is Approved for Use by the FDA—A

Vaccine is approved by the FDA.

Vaccine Safety and Efficacy Supported by Randomized, Controlled, Clinical Trials—C

Safety

Please refer to the discussion of vaccine safety above. As a combination vaccine, it is not possible to distinguish the safety effects of the pertussis vaccine antigens from the diphtheria and tetanus antigens. The inability to distinguish safety signals related to any one antigen represents a major concern about combination vaccines.

As observed with numerous other vaccines on the schedule, control groups never contained true placebos. Control groups in clinical trials for Daptacel® received other vaccines and Infanrix® control groups were either given whole-cell DTP or there was no control group.

The remaining five DTaP brands are combined with other pediatric vaccines such as polio (IPV), hemophilus influenza type B (HIB), and or hepatitis

B (HepB). Safety and vaccine efficacy of these combinations are necessarily confounded by inclusion of multiple distinct vaccines.

For children unable to tolerate the pertussis component or adults who do not need pertussis coverage, there are diphtheria and tetanus (DT) vaccines (generic manufactured by Sanofi) and tetanus and reduced diphtheria vaccines (Td), both generic and Tenivac® brand by Sanofi.

Effectiveness

After three doses of either vaccine, protective efficacy against pertussis infection was around 85%.[36,37] Moreover, raw numbers are not available to estimate Absolute Risk Reduction, which is essential for assessing risk-benefit for the vaccine.

Waning Effectiveness

As noted previously, only 71% of young children have immunity to infection five years after getting their fifth dose of DTaP.[38] The results are worse in adolescents where only 34% have immunity just two to four years after vaccination.[39]

Kaiser Permanente reported that vaccine effectiveness wanes by an average of 27% per year and occurs with all DTaP brands on the market.[40] A 2012 report in the *New England Journal of Medicine* observed that, "after the fifth dose of DTaP, the odds of acquiring pertussis increased by an average of 42% per year."[41]

A review article in *Pediatric Infectious Diseases* examined the development of pertussis vaccines and identified a cause for the sharp decline in acellular vaccine effectiveness. The author cites the relatively small number of antigens presented to the immune system, as the acellular version contains only three to five antigens versus more than three thousand in the whole cell version.[42] Researchers refer to stimulation of the immune system with a limited set of antigens as linked-epitope suppression (an epitope is the part of an antigen to which the immune system attaches an antibody).

In order to mount a strong and durable immune response, multiple antigens derived from several structures of the bacteria or virus are necessary. That is why in most instances, natural immunity is more effective than vaccine-induced immunity. Exposure to the actual pathogen presents the immune system with a complete map of the invader.

The author of the *Pediatric Infectious Diseases* article reaches a pessimistic conclusion:

> Because of linked-epitope suppression, all children who were primed [vaccinated] by DTaP vaccines will be more susceptible to pertussis throughout their lifetimes, and there is no easy way to decrease this increased lifetime susceptibility.[43]

Vaccine Does Not Significantly Impact Developing Childhood Immune, Cardiovascular, Neurological, Hematological, Hormonal, or Musculoskeletal Systems—D

The lack of placebo comparisons, the presence of aluminum compound excipients, and significant reports of adverse events suggest developing organ systems may be at risk of significant impact.

Vaccine Creates Lifelong Immunity—D

Vaccine immunity wanes over time.

Vaccine Important to Reach Herd Immunity—D

The acellular pertussis vaccine does not prevent infection or transmission. As a result, widespread vaccination with DTaP does not create herd immunity for any of the vaccine indications.

Pertussis Overall Grade—C

The risks once again outweigh the benefits in healthy children. DTaP vaccine exposes children to aluminum salts and other toxic excipients, and there is evidence that vaccinated children may become asymptomatic carriers, putting other children at risk. If caregivers are unable to be vigilant for respiratory symptoms in infants, vaccination may be indicated.

Immunocompromised children should be considered high risk from any of these diseases and may derive greater benefit compared with risks than healthy children.

If parents decide to forgo or delay administration of pertussis vaccine, heightened vigilance for signs of respiratory distress is important. These signs may include prolonged cough, congestion, or the classic whoop, where the child has trouble catching his or her breath. Pertussis can be effectively treated with antibiotics if recognized quickly.

Substitution

Although it is difficult to separate out which vaccine component causes a severe reaction, the CDC advises that children who had a "very bad reaction" to DTaP be given DT or Td (lower dose of diphtheria) instead, with the assumption that the pertussis component led to the adverse event. There is no single tetanus vaccine available.

Related Note: CDC Advocates Vaccination During Third Trimester

As noted, infants and young children are the most vulnerable to pertussis infection. The CDC recommends at least three doses to build immunity, given at two, four, and six months. The CDC also recommends Tdap vaccination during mothers' third trimester to protect the infant.

This is all part of a trend by CDC to encourage vaccinations for pregnant women, which at this point include Tdap, RSV, influenza, and COVID-19.[44]

The evidence for the CDC's recommendation will be reviewed, and the risks and benefits of third trimester Tdap will be discussed in Chapter 19, Vaccines and Pregnancy.

CHAPTER 9

Measles, Mumps, Rubella (MMR) Vaccine

MMR stands for measles, mumps, and rubella, three distinct viral diseases that vary widely in symptoms, contagion, transmission, and clinical risk. Even though each disease has a unique vaccine, they were combined into one formulation known as MMR in 1971. A vaccine that combined MMR with varicella (chickenpox), known as MMRV, became available in 2005.

Measles causes a red-bumpy rash that spreads from the face to the feet along with other symptoms like fever, sore throat, and conjunctivitis. It's highly contagious via coughing and sneezing and can be fatal in children.[1]

Mumps is a contagious disease that spreads through direct contact with saliva or respiratory droplets from the mouth, nose, or throat. The disease is best known for puffy cheeks (the result of swollen salivary glands). Some people who get mumps have mild, cold-like symptoms, but most experience fever, headache, muscle aches, fatigue, and loss of appetite.[2]

Rubella (or German measles, which is not related to the measles virus) generally causes a mild illness characterized by low-grade fever, sore throat, and a rash that starts on the face then spreads to the rest of the body. The disease presents the greatest risk to pregnant women and can cause a miscarriage or serious birth defects.[3]

	Measles	Mumps	Rubella
Criteria	**Grade**	**Grade**	**Grade**
Children are at high risk of severe illness or death from disease	**C**	**D**	**D**
Vaccine prevents infection and replication	**A**	**B**	**B**
Vaccine prevents transmission to others	**B**	**B**	**A**
Vaccine is approved for use by the FDA	**A**	**A**	**A**
Vaccine safety and efficacy supported by randomized, controlled, clinical trials	**D**	**C**	**C**

(Continued on next page)

	Measles	Mumps	Rubella
Criteria	**Grade**	**Grade**	**Grade**
Vaccine does not significantly impact developing childhood immune, cardiovascular, neurological, hematological, hormonal, or musculoskeletal systems	**D**	**D**	**D**
Vaccine creates lifelong immunity	**C**	**D**	**C**
Vaccine important to reach herd immunity	**B**	**B**	**A**
Overall Grade	**B**	**C**	**B**

Vaccine Schedule

According to the CDC, the MMR or MMRV vaccine should be administered as a two-dose series at age 12-15 months and age four to six years. The CDC recommends that MMR be administered separately from varicella for dose 1 in children aged 12-47 months.[4]

Vaccines Offered

MMR vaccines are live, attenuated vaccines. There are two standalone MMR vaccines and one combination vaccine available to children in the US.[5] The standalone vaccines are fully interchangeable.[6]

Standalone

Vaccine	Excipients[7]
M-M-R II® (measles, mumps, rubella)	sorbitol, sucrose, hydrolyzed gelatin, recombinant human albumin, neomycin, fetal bovine serum, WI-38 human diploid lung fibroblasts
PRIORIX® (measles, mumps, rubella)	lactose, amino acids, sorbitol, mannitol, bovine serum albumin, and neomycin sulphate

Combination

Vaccine	Excipients[8]
ProQuad® (measles, mumps, rubella, varicella)	MRC-5 cells including DNA and protein, sucrose, hydrolyzed gelatin, sodium chloride, sorbitol, monosodium L-glutamate, sodium phosphate dibasic, recombinant human albumin, sodium bicarbonate, potassium phosphate monobasic, potassium chloride, potassium phosphate dibasic, neomycin, bovine calf serum, other buffer and media ingredients

Contraindications for the standalone and combination vaccines include:[9]

- Severe allergic reaction after a previous dose or to a vaccine component
- Pregnancy
- Known severe immunodeficiency
- Family history of altered immunocompetence

Measles

Criteria	Grade
Children are at high risk of severe illness or death from disease	C
Vaccine prevents infection and replication	A
Vaccine prevents transmission to others	B
Vaccine is approved for use by the FDA	A
Vaccine safety and efficacy supported by randomized, controlled, clinical trials	C
Vaccine does not significantly impact developing childhood immune, cardiovascular, neurological, hematological, hormonal, or musculoskeletal systems	D
Vaccine creates lifelong immunity	C
Vaccine important to reach herd immunity	B
Measles Vaccine Overall Grade	**B**

Children Are at High Risk of Severe Illness or Death from Disease—C

Measles is highly contagious. However, from 1911 to 1962, just before the introduction of the measles vaccine in 1963, the measles case fatality rate dropped from 21 deaths per 1,000 cases to less than 1 death per 1,000 cases.[10] The dramatic improvement in survival is probably related to advancements in living conditions, nutrition, and health care.[11]

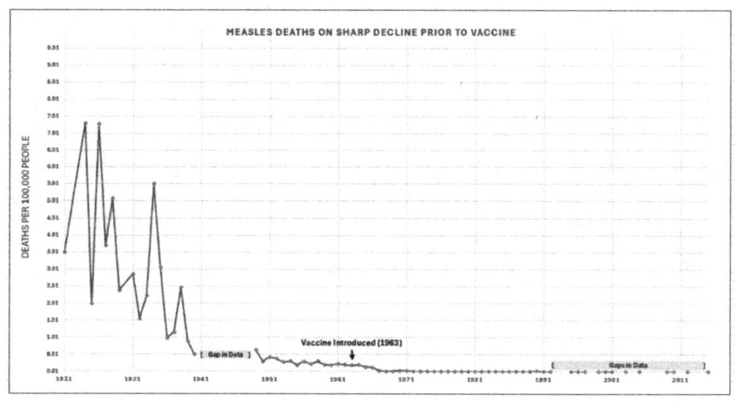

High-risk groups include young children, those with suppressed immune systems, or those who are malnourished and have low levels of Vitamin A. Common complications include ear infections and diarrhea.[12] More serious complications include pneumonia, encephalitis, and something called subacute sclerosing panencephalitis, a rare brain disorder with an onset seven to ten years or more after measles infection.[13]

While the complications noted are concerning, remember that in the modern era, it is rare to suffer permanent disability or death from measles in the US. Although there has been a dramatic decline in the incidence of measles infection since vaccination began, the pre-vaccine mortality rate remains much the same today.

Vaccine Prevents Infection and Replication—A

Vaccine effectively prevents infection and replication.

Vaccine Prevents Transmission to Others—B

Vaccine usually prevents transmission, but there are periodic outbreaks even among immunized children.

Vaccine is Approved for Use by the FDA—A

The vaccine is approved by the FDA.

Vaccine Safety and Efficacy Supported by Randomized, Controlled, Clinical Trials—C

Neither MMR nor its individual component vaccines have ever undergone a randomized controlled clinical trial, and there are no long-term safety studies compared to a placebo.

Safety

According to the CDC, the National Academy of Medicine has determined that

> [E]vidence supports a causal relation between MMR vaccination and anaphylaxis, febrile seizures, thrombocytopenic purpura, transient arthralgia, and measles inclusion body encephalitis in persons with demonstrated immunodeficiencies.[14]

Adverse reactions were recorded for up to forty-two days after vaccination in children with an average age of thirteen months. Reactions after six weeks were not included. Adverse reactions listed in the MMR package insert include:[15]

- Body as a whole: fever; headache; dizziness; malaise; irritability
- Cardiovascular system: vasculitis

- Digestive system: pancreatitis; diarrhea; vomiting; parotitis; nausea
- Hematologic and lymphatic systems: thrombocytopenia; purpura; regional lymphadenopathy; leukocytosis
- Immune system: anaphylaxis, anaphylactoid reactions, angioedema (including peripheral or facial edema) and bronchial spasm
- Musculoskeletal system: arthritis; arthralgia; myalgia
- Nervous system: encephalitis; encephalopathy; measles inclusion body encephalitis (MIBE) subacute sclerosing panencephalitis (SSPE); Guillain-Barré Syndrome (GBS); acute disseminated encephalomyelitis (ADEM); transverse myelitis; febrile convulsions; afebrile convulsions or seizures; ataxia; polyneuritis; polyneuropathy; ocular palsies; paresthesia; syncope
- Respiratory system: pneumonia; pneumonitis; sore throat; cough; rhinitis
- Skin: Stevens-Johnson syndrome; acute hemorrhagic edema of infancy; Henoch-Schönlein purpura; erythema multiforme; urticaria; rash; measles-like rash; pruritus
- Ear: nerve deafness; otitis media
- Eye: retinitis; optic neuritis; papillitis; conjunctivitis
- Urogenital system: epididymitis; orchitis

The rate of occurrence for each of these adverse events is not disclosed.

MMR and Autism Spectrum Disorder

It is generally accepted in the medical community, and it is the CDC's unequivocal position, that vaccines do not cause autism, which is actually a component of Autism Spectrum Disorder, or ASD.[16] Chapter 10, MMR and ASD, critically examines the evidence put forward by the CDC in support of its position and discusses recent analyses that have challenged the CDC's position. In view of the rising incidence of autism in the US, it is vital to understand the potential role of childhood vaccines.

Efficacy

According to the CDC, two doses of MMR vaccine are about 97% effective at preventing measles; one dose is about 93% effective. Widespread use of measles virus-containing vaccines has led to a greater than 99% reduction in measles cases compared with the pre-vaccine era.[17]

The source of the CDC's effectiveness claim is not disclosed. The current vaccine M-M-R II® package insert and the manufacturer's website indicate the vaccine has only been studied for antibody responses to antigens as measured by blood tests and not for actual clinical effectiveness.[18,19]

As a result, estimates of vaccine Relative Risk Reduction and Absolute Risk Reduction are not possible for infection, severity, hospitalization, or death for measles, mumps, or rubella. This does not mean they are not effective, but it does mean that it is difficult to counsel patients regarding their individual risk reduction.

Waning Immunity

Immunity from measles vaccination is known to wane over time.[20] Measles outbreaks continue to occur in highly vaccinated regions and low measles exposure settings.[21] Of great concern is the emergence of measles in infants born to vaccinated mothers. The measles attack rate in children under fifteen months is nearly triple that of babies born to unvaccinated mothers.[22]

For example, in the first four months of 2019, a period when about two thirds of measles cases had already been reported for the year, 25% of cases were in children under fifteen months of age.[23] Ordinarily, mothers with natural immunity to measles pass along strong antibody protection to their infants for the first twelve months of life. Studies of neutralizing antibodies in infants found that children born to naturally immune mothers were more than three times as likely to have protective antibodies at eight months as children of immunized mothers.[24]

In other words, children born to immunized mothers are at much greater risk of measles infection before their first immunization. The very young and adults whose immunity has waned are at much greater risk of serious complications such as pneumonia and encephalitis.

Unfortunately, a third dose of MMR vaccine in young adults provides no additional immune benefit.[25] As with mumps and rubella, natural immunity to measles has proven to be more robust and enduring.

Possible Protective Effect of Measles Infection

Numerous studies have found correlations between measles infection and protection against certain cancers as well as Parkinson's disease in adulthood. Cancers include lymphatic cancers, Hodgkin's disease, non-Hodgkin's lymphoma, and GI, lung, and ENT cancers.[26,27,28,29,30] The degree of protection for each of these cancers is not known and confirmation requires additional studies.

Vaccine Does Not Significantly Impact Developing Childhood Immune, Cardiovascular, Neurological, Hematological, Hormonal, or Musculoskeletal Systems—D

The extensive list of adverse events without CDC disclosure of the rate of occurrence raises concerns about the impact on developing childhood systems.

Vaccine Creates Lifelong Immunity—C

Immunity is known to wane over time and outbreaks are reported periodically.

Vaccine Important to Reach Herd Immunity—B

MMR blocks transmission, but unlike natural immunity, duration of immunity is unknown.

Measles Vaccine Overall Grade—B

Vaccination has dramatically reduced the incidence of measles infections but has had little impact on mortality. Post-approval adverse events suggest vaccination can result in serious disabilities. Lack of vaccine comparison with a placebo, and the absence of Relative Risk Reduction and Absolute Risk Reduction data, makes individual risk assessment difficult.

Potential risks may not outweigh benefits in healthy children. Measles infections are generally mild to moderate in childhood, but across millions of children will result in some hospitalizations and deaths, particularly in children with chronic illnesses.

However, measles infections need to be compared with the potential long-term risks of MMR vaccines. These include allergies, autoimmune and neurodevelopmental disorders during childhood, and the potential for severe infections due to waning effectiveness during adulthood. Knowledge about the full range of long-term health effects of MMR in comparison with the benefits for millions of children is simply incomplete.

As a result, individual risk should be considered as opposed to blanket immunization for measles vaccinations. Those at high risk, such as chronically ill or immunocompromised children may gain the greatest benefit compared to risks, whereas risks may outweigh benefits in healthy children or those who have had the disease.

Alternatively, caregivers might consider delaying initial MMR vaccination in healthy children after the scheduled twelve to fifteen months to give the child's brain and other developing systems time to develop before powerful, artificial immune system stimulation from multiple vaccines.

Mumps

Criteria	Grade
Children are at high risk of severe illness or death from disease	**D**
Vaccine prevents infection and replication	**B**
Vaccine prevents transmission to others	**B**
Vaccine is approved for use by the FDA	**A**
Vaccine safety and efficacy supported by randomized, controlled, clinical trials	**C**
Vaccine does not significantly impact developing childhood immune, cardiovascular, neurological, hematological, hormonal, or musculoskeletal systems	**D**

(Continued on next page)

Criteria	Grade
Vaccine creates lifelong immunity	D
Vaccine important to reach herd immunity	B
Mumps Vaccine Overall Grade	**C**

Children Are at High Risk of Severe Illness or Death From Disease—D

Most children have mild symptoms or none at all. According to the CDC, mumps can occasionally cause complications, especially in adults.[31] Complications can include inflammation of the testes, ovaries, pancreas, and brain.

Vaccine Prevents Infection and Replication—B

Vaccine prevents infection and replication, but periodic outbreaks in vaccinated persons indicate breakthrough infections do occur.

Vaccine Prevents Transmission to Others—B

Clinical studies examined antibody responses to vaccination and not clinical outcomes. Therefore, Relative Risk Reduction and Absolute Risk Reduction are not known. The marked reduction in cases following vaccination indicates the vaccine is effective at preventing infection, replication, and transmission.

However, waning immunity and occasional outbreaks in vaccinated persons indicate transmission to others does occur in vaccinated persons.

Vaccine is Approved For Use by the FDA—A

The vaccine is approved by the FDA.

Vaccine Safety and Efficacy Supported by Randomized, Controlled, Clinical Trials—C

Safety

When it comes to combination vaccines, it is difficult to separate out a safety signal (statistical evidence that the vaccine may cause a serious adverse event) for any particular antigen. See the safety section under Vaccine Safety and Efficacy for measles (p. 84).

Effectiveness

According to the CDC, the mumps component of the MMR vaccine is about 88% effective when a person gets two doses; one dose is about 78% effective. Since the pre-vaccine era, there has been more than a 99% decrease in mumps cases in the United States, largely due to herd immunity from MMR vaccine.[32]

Waning Immunity

Mumps immunity from vaccination is known to wane over time. Following decades of decline and widespread vaccination, outbreaks of mumps have occurred in the US and other developed countries. For example:

2016—Harvard mumps outbreak grows; dozens infected; all students affected had been immunized against mumps.[33]

2014—Mumps outbreak hits Fordham University; all students diagnosed with mumps had been vaccinated.[34]

2014—Stevens Institute of Technology reports 8 cases, despite students having been fully vaccinated.[35]

Analysis of data from multiple studies estimates that immune protection against mumps wanes on average 27 years post-vaccination, putting people in their thirties at risk if exposed.[36] This has prompted calls for a third dose of MMR at 18 years or boosters throughout adulthood.

Mumps in adulthood can be life threatening and can include complications such as meningitis, encephalitis, orchitis (inflammation of the testicle), pancreatitis, and deafness. Of course, the risk of infection during adulthood and a call for boosters would be unnecessary for healthy adults who acquired immunity naturally during childhood.

Vaccine Does Not Significantly Impact Developing Childhood Immune, Cardiovascular, Neurological, Hematological, Hormonal, or Musculoskeletal Systems—D

See discussion under measles (p. 86).

Vaccine Creates Lifelong Immunity—D

Waning immunity and regular outbreaks among vaccinated students and others indicates many do not have lifelong immunity.

Vaccine Important to Reach Herd Immunity—B

MMR blocks transmission, but unlike natural immunity, duration of immunity is unknown.

Mumps Vaccine Overall Grade—C

Vaccination has dramatically reduced the incidence of mumps infections, generally a mild disease in healthy kids. Waning effectiveness and periodic outbreaks raise the possibility of increased risk of infection during adulthood when the disease is much more dangerous.

Post-approval adverse events suggest vaccination can result in serious disabilities. These include allergies, autoimmune and neurodevelopmental disorders during childhood, and the potential for severe infections due to waning effectiveness during adulthood.

Knowledge about the full range of long-term health effects of MMR in comparison with the benefits for millions of children is simply incomplete. Lack of vaccine comparison with a placebo and the absence of Relative Risk Reduction and Absolute Risk Reduction data makes individual risk assessment difficult. As a result, individual risk should be considered as opposed to blanket immunization for mumps vaccinations. Those at high risk, such as chronically ill or immunocompromised children, may gain the greatest benefit compared to risks.

In healthy children, risks likely outweigh benefits during early childhood. Caregivers might consider delaying initial MMR vaccination in healthy children until after the scheduled twelve to fifteen months to give the child's brain and other immature systems time to develop before powerful, artificial immune system stimulation from multiple vaccines.

Rubella

Criteria	Grade
Children are at high risk of severe illness or death from disease	D
Vaccine prevents infection and replication	B
Vaccine prevents transmission to others	A
Vaccine is approved for use by the FDA	A
Vaccine safety and efficacy supported by randomized, controlled, clinical trials	C
Vaccine does not significantly impact developing childhood immune, cardiovascular, neurological, hematological, hormonal, or musculoskeletal systems	D
Vaccine creates lifelong immunity	C
Vaccine important to reach herd immunity	A
Rubella Vaccine Overall Grade	**B**

Children Are at High Risk of Severe Illness or Death from Disease—D

Rubella symptoms in children are usually mild, and up to 50% of infections may be asymptomatic.[37] Infection confers lifelong immunity. The greatest risk is to pregnant women during their first fifteen to twenty weeks of pregnancy, when it can infect the fetus.

Fetal disease is known as congenital rubella syndrome (CRS) and can cause a range of complications from miscarriage to fetal death to developmental abnormalities. As such, it is vital that women of child-bearing years be protected.

Therefore, the main objective of rubella vaccination is to prevent congenital rubella syndrome that can lead to miscarriages, stillbirths, and birth defects.

Vaccine Prevents Infection and Replication—B

The vaccine prevents infection and replication in the vast majority of cases; however, waning immunity has been described. See Vaccine Safety and Efficacy below.

Vaccine Prevents Transmission to Others—A

Largely as a result of vaccination, rubella was eliminated from the US in 2004. Less than ten cases occur each year in persons who have been living or traveling abroad.[38]

Vaccine is Approved for Use by the FDA—A

The vaccine is approved by the FDA.

Vaccine Safety and Efficacy Supported by Randomized, Controlled, Clinical Trials—C

Safety

For combination vaccines, it is difficult to separate out a safety signal (statistical evidence that the vaccine may cause a serious adverse event) for any particular antigen. See the Safety section under Vaccine Safety and Effectiveness for measles (p. 84).

Efficacy

According to antibody studies, one dose of the MMR vaccine is 98% effective at preventing rubella, and maintains that level of prevention after two doses.[39] Prior to the availability of the MMR vaccine, rubella was a common disease in the US, although not as widespread as measles and mumps.

The current vaccine M-M-R II® package insert and the manufacturer's website indicate the vaccine has only been studied for antibody responses to antigens as measured by blood tests and not for actual clinical effectiveness.[40,41]

As a result, estimates of vaccine Relative Risk Reduction and Absolute Risk Reduction are not possible for infection, severity, hospitalization, or death for measles, mumps, or rubella. This does not mean they are not effective, but it does mean that it is difficult to counsel patients regarding their individual risk reduction.

Waning Immunity

A single dose of MMR vaccine is said to confer lifelong immunity to rubella. However, some women will fail to develop protective rubella antibody levels. As such, early vaccination may provide a false sense of security.

Women immunized at a younger age (fifteen months) were less likely to develop protective antibodies relative to women who were vaccinated later in childhood.[42]

For women who have received a single dose of MMR, a second dose is recommended before onset of childbearing years.

Vaccine Does Not Significantly Impact Developing Childhood Immune, Cardiovascular, Neurological, Hematological, Hormonal, or Musculoskeletal Systems—D

See discussion under measles (p. 87).

Vaccine Creates Lifelong Immunity—C

See discussion above under Waning Immunity (p. 92).

Vaccine Important to Reach Herd Immunity—A

Rubella has been virtually eliminated in the US since 2004.

Rubella Vaccine Overall Grade—B

The rubella vaccine risk-benefit profile is distinct from measles and mumps vaccines. Of the three diseases MMR is intended to prevent, rubella poses a disproportionate health risk as noted above. Every effort should be made to avoid rubella infection during pregnancy.

MMR presents a risk profile that has been minimized by the CDC. The actual risk to childhood immune, neurological, hematological, and other developing systems is likely significant. However, the true incidence has been obscured by the failure to compare vaccine adverse events against true placebos.

For parents and caregivers who elect to withhold or defer administration of MMR until later in childhood, consideration should be given to immunize girls during elementary school and again after the onset of menses to help assure the development of protective antibodies prior to pregnancy. Unfortunately, there is no single rubella vaccine and vaccination requires the combined MMR vaccine.

> If there is any doubt about the level of protection, all women who are or may become pregnant should be tested for the presence of rubella IgG antibody levels sufficient to confer immunity. Inadequate levels can be remedied through MMR vaccination.

CHAPTER 10

MMR and Autism Spectrum Disorder (ASD)—The Great Debate

"Linking vaccines to autism is the third rail of public health, touch it at your peril."

—E. Y. Davis, MD

In 1995, ASD was diagnosed in 1 in 1000 US children. By 2000, the ratio surged to 1 in 150, and 20 years later an estimated 1 in 36 children have ASD. Autism is a subset of ASD. A diagnosis of ASD includes several conditions including autistic disorder, Asperger syndrome, and pervasive developmental disorder, also called atypical autism.

Why the Rise?

There have been many attempts to explain the dramatic rise in the disorder, most notably improved screening, increased awareness, and access to services by the underserved. At least two studies, including one by the state of California, dispute these factors as principal reasons for the exploding number of cases.

Year	CDC Schedule	Autism Rates
1983	10 vaccines	1 in 10,000
2013	32 vaccines	1 in 88
2018	74 vaccines	1 in 36

A 300% rise in ASD over 20 years warrants a look at other potential contributing factors. These might include diet, pollution, environmental toxins, social media, declining social interaction, lack of exercise, pharmaceuticals, and vaccines.

"Vaccines Do Not Cause Autism"—CDC

CDC cites several studies and reviews by expert panels in support of their position. The agency claims the evidence is consistent and overwhelming that ASD is a neurodevelopmental disability unaffected by vaccination. In other words, you're "born with it."

Any challenge to this position, held by virtually every national authoritative body on vaccines and ASD, is considered heretical and beyond discussion. Just Google "vaccines and autism" and the consensus of the Big Pharma-Government-Industrial complex will become clear.

Recent experience suggests a healthy dose of skepticism about declarations by the CDC is warranted. The nation has just been through a pandemic where most CDC, NIH, FDA, Big Pharma, and Academy dogma about COVID-19 prevention and treatment have proven either false, exaggerated, or downright dangerous.

See Chapter 4, COVID-19 and Chapter 17, Why Your Child Should Never, Ever Be Given an mRNA Vaccine for additional details.

Vaccine-Autism Research

A close look at the key studies the CDC cites as support for denial of a link between ASD and vaccines reveals considerable uncertainty. The data is not as clear-cut as the public has been led to believe and, in some cases, contradicts the conclusions. To assert that vaccines have been studied for their role in autism is simply misleading.

What the Studies Reveal

By the time a child living in the US reaches twelve months, he/she will have received twenty-six vaccines, up to six at a time–more than any other country in the world. Other than MMR, none of the remaining twenty-three have been evaluated for an association with ASD. MMR stands alone as the only vaccine that has been evaluated with respect to a link with autism.

On its face, the CDC's assertion that vaccines as a category do not cause autism is demonstrably false. It is equally true that no link has been proven, but there are warning signs everywhere if you look for them.

Vaccines Contain More Than Just Weakened, Killed, or Parts of Viruses

In addition to antigens (components of a virus, bacteria, or other pathogen that trigger an immune response), vaccines contain a number of additives called excipients (see Chapter 2, Do No Harm). According to the CDC, there are thirty-eight separate ingredients present in two or more vaccines on the schedule.

Only a single excipient, thimerosal, has been examined for a link with ASD.

Thimerosal has largely been eliminated from most vaccines (still present in lesser amounts in some flu vaccines) due to concerns about neurotoxicity, but there are thirty-seven other excipients that have not been studied for their potential to cause ASD. Several have known toxicity, including aluminum salts, formaldehyde, and polysorbate 80. These ingredients are rarely even mentioned in the studies that dismiss a vaccine-autism link.

CDC Evidence against a Link Between Vaccines and Autism

A handful of studies frame the core argument that dismisses a vaccine-autism association. Two of these studies, by Jain et al and Taylor et al, are frequently cited and are representative of the prevailing thinking on the topic.

Jain et al: Autism Occurrence by MMR Vaccine Status among US Children With Older Siblings With and Without Autism

This study has served as the darling of the mainstream media and is frequently cited in the medical literature as proof that vaccines do not cause autism. However, the study is seriously flawed.

Author Conflicts of Interest

Five of the six authors are employed by the Lewin Group or its parent, Optum, a large PR/health-care consulting firm whose clients include the federal government and some of the largest vaccine makers in the world.

Regarding the study itself, there are numerous methodological weaknesses. The authors claim to have compared vaccinated with unvaccinated children, as noted in this 2019 press release on the study:

> In all, the researchers analyzed the health records of 95,727 children, including more than 15,000 children unvaccinated at age 2 and more than 8,000 still unvaccinated at age 5.[1]

But . . . Did Jain Have an Unvaccinated Control Group?

Upon closer examination, "unvaccinated" was the term applied when study authors could not identify if the child had received the MMR vaccine through insurance claims data. It did *not* mean the child was otherwise unvaccinated. Nor did it mean children in the control group never received the MMR vaccine if it was not submitted as an insurance claim.

For example, they could have been vaccinated at school, a health fair, or a local clinic without filing a claim. This idea is reinforced by the study, which reported a lower rate of MMR vaccination compared with national rates. As the study authors note:

> The MMR immunization rates in our study were 4% to 14% lower than rates reported in the National Immunization Survey. Thus, children in our study who are considered unvaccinated may have received vaccines in settings such as schools or public health clinics in which claims were not submitted.[2]

A vaccinated control group is hardly a control group. These are glaring study weaknesses that call into question the authors' conclusions.

Taylor et al: Vaccines Are Not Associated With Autism. An Evidence-based Meta-analysis of Case-control and Cohort Studies

Taylor et al is a meta-analysis of ten previous studies, six of which are MMR-related. A meta-analysis is the statistical combination of results from two or more separate studies, and in this case it was concluded that vaccines are not associated with autism.[3]

Critique of Taylor Analysis

There are several weaknesses in the underlying studies analyzed by Taylor. For example, three of the studies show an apparent protective effect of MMR vaccines against autism, ranging from 8-83%. In other words, children who received vaccines were less likely to develop autism.

The presence of a protective effect of vaccines over placebo suggests selection bias in the study groups. An unbiased study purporting to demonstrate no difference in the incidence of autism between MMR and unvaccinated children should not show any significant difference, positive or negative, in the rate of autism.

Identification of a protective effect could mean either that the vaccine group enrolled children at lower risk than the placebo control group or that children in the control group were more likely to develop autism. Either way, the study results are suspect.

DeStefano Study

One of the six MMR studies cited by Taylor et al was authored by Drs. deStefano and Thomspon and published in the journal *Pediatrics* in 2004. The authors conclude:

> The evidence now is convincing that the measles-mumps-rubella vaccine does not cause autism or any particular subtypes of autistic spectrum disorder.[4]

After publication, the second author, Dr. William Thompson, publicly denounced the study conclusions. He wrote:

> I regret that my coauthors and I omitted statistically significant information in our 2004 article published in the journal Pediatrics. The omitted data suggested that African American males who received the MMR vaccine before age 36 months were at increased risk for autism. Decisions were made regarding which findings to report after the data were collected, and I believe that the final study protocol was not followed.[5]

Such a public repudiation by an author of a study published in a mainstream medical journal is rare. The statement implies there may be a safety signal from MMR vaccination in African American male children that is being ignored.

DeStefano Study Reassessed

This "confession" by Thompson led one researcher (Hooker) unrelated to the original team to reanalyze the study data. What he discovered was quite the opposite of the original authors' conclusions. His reanalysis, published in 2018, found a strong, statistically significant relationship between MMR vaccine and autism.

Hooker concludes:

> The first data set used by DeStefano et.al represents a huge lost opportunity to understand any role between the timing of the first MMR vaccine and autism. The re-analysis presented here elucidates effects that should at least merit further investigation. Specifically, increased risks of earlier vaccination are observed for African American males and among cases of autism without MR [mental retardation]. Both phenomena deserve additional study that could yield important clues regarding the current enormous increase in autism. [6]

Madsen et al. Study

Another MMR study cited by Taylor et al was performed in Denmark and included over 500,000 children.[7] Several factors mitigate against the authors' conclusion that their study makes a strong argument against a causal relation between MMR vaccination and autism.

First, it is an observational study that looks back on data coded into a national registry rather than a prospective trial. The main problems with observational studies is selection bias and the presence of confounders (unaccounted for variables), both of which are prevented in a randomized, controlled clinical trial.

One of the confounders in an observational study of vaccines is something called healthy vaccinee bias, where healthy persons are more likely to get vaccinated, thereby skewing the results.[8] Healthy vaccinee bias can not be ruled out in Madsen et al.

Similar to many of the vaccine clinical trials, Madsen et al fail to have a control group that received no vaccines for comparison. Even if a Danish child failed to receive the MMR vaccine, many would have gotten DTaP, IPV and Hib by the time MMR was administered. The assumption that none of those nor the excipients they contain are causally related to the onset of ASD is simply unproven.

Another factor unaccounted for is the onset of ASD symptoms prior to a diagnosis. A prior diagnosis was an exclusion criterion for the study. But symptoms typically emerge over months to years prior to a diagnosis. Parents concerned about ASD symptoms may be less likely to vaccinate their children, which could bias the sample.

This latter factor may well have been exacerbated by restrictions on who can record an ASD diagnosis in Denmark. The Madsen study notes that "[o]nly specialists in child and adolescent psychiatry are authorized to code the diagnosis of autism in the Danish Psychiatric Central Register.[9]

So a child couldn't even obtain a diagnosis of ASD that was entered into the Danish Psychiatric Central Register until they could be seen by a specialist in Psychiatry. Moreover, children on the lower end of the Spectrum may not have been seen by a psychiatrist, leading to undercounting of ASD.

As the authors noted, "Reporting of the other autistic-spectrum disorders is less complete than that for autistic disorders, and some diagnoses are almost certainly missed."[10] They go on to state, "Our records did not contain information on when the first autistic symptoms were noted, and we could not adjust for a differential delay in the diagnosis."[11]

Then there is this unfortunate detail: The Madsen study coordinator working on behalf of the CDC is wanted in the US for financial fraud for misappropriating autism research funds for his personal use. Notably, the US government appears to show no interest in extraditing him back to the US.

A follow-up Danish study published in 2019 by one of Madsen's coauthors claims to reinforce Madsen et al. and other studies that find, "MMR vaccination does not increase the risk for autism, does not trigger autism in susceptible children . . . "[12] Although there were improvements in study methodology since Madsen's publication, similar factors undermine the conclusions reached.

These include an observational study design, lack of an unvaccinated control group, MMR injections that follow other standard vaccinations, and potential delays in diagnosis of ASD. One study critic noted that a more accurate conclusion for the study might be, "Later MMR vaccination does not increase the risk in comparison to a cocktail of previously administered vaccines."[13]

Two other potential confounding factors are noted. First, financial support for the study was provided by the Danish Ministry of Health and the Novo Nordisk Foundation. The latter Foundation is an investor in vaccine development and owns a controlling interest in the Danish pharmaceutical company Novo Nordisk.[14]

In addition, two of the editors of the journal that published the study have ownership in major pharmaceutical companies.[15] These examples don't in themselves prove a conflict of interest, but serve as a reminder of the close relationship that exists between industry, government, and research organizations.

A meta-analysis is only as good as the reliability of the data in the underlying studies. With that in mind, Taylor et al.'s conclusions remain open to debate.

Comparisons with Unvaccinated Children Needed

A comparison of outcomes between vaccinated and truly unvaccinated children, something missing from Taylor's analysis, helps to inform the debate.

Fortunately, such investigations exist. After publication of the Taylor et al and Jain et al papers, two studies were published in 2017 by Mawson et al that compared vaccinated with completely unvaccinated, home-schooled children.

The studies shared a common dataset but were separated into two analyses due to some startling findings.

The first study looked at children born at term and the second study looked at children born prematurely. The results were so significant and so contrary to prevailing opinion that the media refused to cover it.

Vaccinated children were found to have a nearly four-fold higher incidence of autism than the unvaccinated. Mawson concluded:

> The vaccinated were less likely than the unvaccinated to have been diagnosed with chickenpox and pertussis, but more likely to have been diagnosed with pneumonia, otitis media, allergies and NDD [neurodevelopmental disorders]. After adjustment, vaccination, male gender, and preterm birth remained significantly associated with NDD.[16]

Premature Infants at Extreme Risk

Results from Mawson's second study that included premature children were even more devastating. Children born prematurely and vaccinated were five times more likely to develop a neurodevelopmental disorder than unvaccinated preterm infants and fourteen times more likely to develop a neurodevelopmental disorder compared with unvaccinated, term infants.

Mawson found no association between prematurity and autism except after vaccination. The authors concluded:

> Preterm birth coupled with vaccination, however, was associated with a synergistic increase in the odds of NDD, suggesting the possibility that vaccination could precipitate adverse neurodevelopmental outcomes in preterm infants. These results provide clues to the epidemiology and causation of NDD but question the safety of current vaccination programs for preterm infants.[17]

There are important caveats about the Mawson studies. They are authored by a single research group, the sample size was relatively small (666 total, although most results achieved statistical significance), the study has not been replicated with a larger sample size (due to limitation of funding), data collection was based on a questionnaire completed by mothers of the children, and no chart reviews were performed.

Despite these shortcomings, Mawson raises legitimate concerns about the effect of vaccination of neurodevelopmental disorders.

Nationwide Study of Childhood Vaccination and Autism

A nationwide study by Delong examined the relationship between the proportion of children who received the recommended vaccines by age two years and the prevalence of autism and speech or language impairment.[18] The study reported a positive and statistically significant relationship between vaccination and neurodevelopmental delays.

How Vaccines or Excipients Might Cause Autism

Many theories exist. One is that vaccinations create inflammation in the brain similar to what has been observed in autistic brains. Some studies have linked this inflammation to aluminum and the measles virus component of the MMR vaccine.

For example, vaccine measles virus was observed to correlate with the production of autoantibodies to brain tissue.[19] This means the immune system may be switched on to attack normal brain tissue after MMR vaccination. Measles antibodies were found to be significantly higher in autistic children, but not antibodies to mumps or rubella.[20]

Evidence for Brain Inflammation

Evidence for brain injury post-measles vaccination comes from a review of cases submitted to the National Vaccine Injury Compensation Program.[21] Measles-only vaccines (pre-combination with mumps and rubella) are linked to severe brain injury and death.

A total of forty-eight children developed encephalopathy (brain injury and damage) within fifteen days of vaccination where no other cause could be identified. Eight children died, and the remainder had mental regression and retardation, chronic seizures, motor and sensory deficits, and movement disorders.[22]

A newborn generates one million neural synapses per second, making neural circuitry extremely vulnerable to toxic insults.[23] This is why it may make sense to consider delaying and/or spacing out vaccinations or eliminating some of them altogether during this vulnerable period, depending on a child's particular risk profile.

Summary of Research on MMR and Autism

Based on the available information, the relationship of MMR vaccination or any of its excipients to autism has neither been proven nor disproven. The CDC has failed to make its case that vaccines do not cause autism.

Unfortunately, the Big Pharma-Government-Industrial complex is so compromised by self-interest that it is inconceivable to expect NIH, NIAID, or CDC to conduct objective studies of the relationship of ASD to either vaccines or excipients.

Pre-Covid-19, the US vaccine industry was $30 billion per year, growing at 10% per year. The pace of growth has accelerated post-COVID-19, as have all the interests that rely on the vaccine juggernaut, both political and economic.

Finding problems with vaccines is not a research funding priority. Just look at COVID-19 vaccines. They don't prevent infection, replication, or transmission.

They rapidly develop negative vaccine efficacy against hospitalization and death. Yet they are still being aggressively promoted.

Challenges to this industry come with great peril, especially to those dependent on federal research grants or pharmaceutical company funding.

PART THREE

The Remaining Six Considered

CHAPTER 11

Varicella (Chickenpox) Vaccine

Chickenpox is a mild disease in most children, producing fever, headache, sore throat, stomachache, and a blistering, itchy rash. This viral infection rarely causes serious illness except in those with chronic illness or weakened immune systems. Death from chickenpox is extremely rare and mostly occurs in adults. Infection confers lifelong immunity, although all who are infected are at risk of delayed herpes zoster infection (shingles). Prior to the 1990s, chickenpox infection was an ordinary childhood experience. Nearly every American born before 1980 had chickenpox, even if they don't remember it.

Vaccination effectively reduces the incidence of a generally mild disease, but the duration of immunity remains in question. In contrast, immunity from infection is lifelong. Widespread varicella immunization may paradoxically underlie the rising incidence of shingles, especially in those under sixty.

In 1995, the CDC added chickenpox vaccine to the childhood vaccine schedule for 12–15-month-olds in an effort to eliminate the minor risk of hospitalization or death and to protect those who were at elevated risk. Adoption of the varicella vaccine was not universal. Several western countries such as Austria, Belgium, France, Denmark and Portugal considered the risk versus benefit of vaccination did not justify a vaccine requirement and hold that position to this day.

Criteria	Grade
Children are at high risk of severe illness or death from disease	**D**
Vaccine prevents infection and replication	**B**
Vaccine prevents transmission to others	**B**
Vaccine is approved for use by the FDA	**A**
Vaccine safety and efficacy supported by randomized, controlled, clinical trials	**C**

(Continued on next page)

Criteria	Grade
Vaccine does not significantly impact developing childhood immune, cardiovascular, neurological, hematological, hormonal, or musculoskeletal systems	B
Vaccine creates lifelong immunity	C
Vaccine important to achieve herd immunity	B
Overall Grade	B

Vaccine Schedule

The CDC recommends that all children receive two doses of the varicella vaccine. The first dose is administered between 12-15 months of age and the second at 4-6 years old.[1]

Vaccines Offered

Varicella vaccine is a live, attenuated virus vaccine, meaning the virus is chemically treated to keep it from replicating once injected, although transmission of varicella vaccine virus has been reported.[2] There are two versions of varicella vaccine approved in the US.

Standalone

Vaccine	Excipients[3]
Varivax® (single-antigen varicella vaccine)	sucrose, hydrolyzed gelatin, sodium chloride, monosodium L-glutamate, sodium phosphate dibasic, potassium phosphate monobasic, potassium chloride, MRC-5 human diploid cells including DNA & protein, sodium phosphate monobasic, EDTA, neomycin, fetal bovine serum

Combination

Vaccine	Excipients[4]
ProQuad® (measles, mumps, rubella, and varicella)	MRC-5 cells including DNA and protein, sucrose, hydrolyzed gelatin, sodium chloride, sorbitol, monosodium L-glutamate, sodium phosphate dibasic, recombinant human albumin, sodium bicarbonate, potassium phosphate monobasic, potassium chloride, potassium phosphate dibasic, neomycin, bovine calf serum, other buffer and media ingredients

The list of contraindications is long. The vaccine should be avoided by anyone who:[5]

- has a history of anaphylactic/anaphylactoid reaction to gelatin, neomycin, or any other component of the vaccine.
- has blood dyscrasias, leukemia, lymphomas, or malignant neoplasms affecting bone marrow or the lymphatic system.
- has a primary or acquired immunodeficiency, including persons with immunosuppression associated with cellular immunodeficiencies and AIDS or severe immunosuppression associated with HIV infection.
- is receiving prolonged, high-dose systemic immunosuppressive therapy (≥2 weeks), including large doses of oral steroids (≥2mg/kg of body weight or a total of 20mg/day of prednisone or its equivalent for people who weigh >10kg) or other immunosuppressive therapy.
- has a moderate or severe concurrent illness.
- has a family history (first degree relatives) of congenital hereditary immunodeficiency, unless the person has been determined to be immunocompetent.
- is or may be pregnant.

Children Are at High Risk of Severe Illness or Death from Disease—D

Chickenpox is usually a mild disease in healthy children. Immunocompromised children without evidence of immunity and those infected during the first twelve months when they are not eligible for the vaccine are at greatest risk of severe illness.

Vaccine Prevents Infection and Replication—B

Two doses of the vaccine effectively prevent infection and replication during childhood at around 98%, although the Absolute Risk Reduction is closer to 33%.[6] Absolute Risk Reduction in this instance means that for any vaccinated child, the risk of infection is reduced by 33%, not 98% compared with an unvaccinated child.

See Chapter 2, Do No Harm, for further discussion about the important distinction between Absolute Risk Reduction versus Relative Risk Reduction when discussing vaccine efficacy.

A study from 2019 reports that vaccination cut the rates of rare herpes zoster (shingles) infections in children by 78%. However, in terms of absolute risk reduction, the rate was only cut by 0.1%.[7] This means that for any particular child, their risk of getting zoster is reduced by just 0.1% after vaccination, reflecting the rarity of the disease in children. Shingles in children is largely restricted to the immunocompromised and those infected with the chickenpox during the first year of life.

The duration of immunity, although most likely a decade or more, remains uncertain as the two-vaccination schedule has only been in place since 2006.

Vaccine Prevents Transmission to Others—B

Fully immunized children are highly unlikely to pass the virus on to others during childhood. However, reliable prevention of transmission after ten years remains uncertain.

Vaccine is Approved for Use by the FDA—A

The vaccines are approved by the FDA.

Vaccine Safety and Efficacy Supported by Randomized, Controlled, Clinical Trials—C

Safety Testing

The current refrigerated varicella vaccine, Varivax®, has not been subjected to randomized, controlled clinical trials, so absent a placebo control group there is no reliable long-term safety data. In one study of a predecessor vaccine, two different concentrations of the same vaccine antigens (immune system stimulants) were compared with each other. Other studies have compared a one-dose versus a two-dose regimen.[8]

A true placebo injection would not contain anything other than an innocuous substance such as saline. On the other hand, if the placebo contains active ingredients, then side effects from the placebo itself could mask the rate of complications in the test group when the two groups are compared.

The vaccine was never tested for carcinogenesis, mutagenesis, or impact on fertility.

Efficacy

In 2006, the CDC added a second booster dose for four- to six-year-old children due to waning effectiveness of a single dose. One dose of vaccine was shown to protect roughly 85% of children, increasing to 98% protection after a second dose was administered. As noted above, the Absolute Risk Reduction is closer to 33% for any particular child.

Natural immunity from chickenpox infection, as with other previously common childhood communicable viral diseases like mumps, measles, and rubella, confers lifelong immunity. Breakthrough infection is rare.

Waning Efficacy

The evidence is conflicting about waning vaccine effectiveness. According to the CDC:

> It is not known how long a vaccinated person is protected against varicella. But live vaccines in general provide long-lasting immunity. Several studies have shown that people vaccinated against varicella had antibodies for at least ten to 20 years after vaccination.[9] [It bears repeating that antibody studies are not the equivalent of disease prevention.]

As per the package insert,

> The duration of protection of VARIVAX® is unknown; however, long-term efficacy studies have demonstrated continued protection up to ten years after vaccination.[10,11]

If varicella vaccination is like other childhood vaccines, effectiveness will inevitably wane for most. Waning immunity has the potential to infect adults at higher risk of complications. There is no evidence (yet) that waning immunity is increasing rates of reinfection in adults, but it's only been eighteen years since introduction of the booster vaccine in 2006.

The implications of waning immunity from infection are significant. These include the risk of infection during adulthood when the illness can be severe, infection during pregnancy, and the occurrence of herpes zoster eruption (shingles).

Varicella infection in pregnant women is dangerous to both the mother and fetus, including fetal varicella syndrome (FVS) and varicella infection of the newborn, which comprises congenital varicella syndrome (CVS) and neonatal varicella. Infection in adults can lead to potentially lethal viral pneumonia, encephalitis, septicemia (infection in the blood), and toxic shock syndrome. Healthy adults with natural immunity are not generally at risk of any of these conditions, except for shingles in those over sixty. As will be discussed, the rising incidence of shingles in adults under sixty years of age may be an indication of waning vaccine protection.

It is also possible that vaccinated adults with waning immunity may be protected by herd immunity in the vaccinated population at large. Or perhaps insufficient time has passed to surface all the effects of waning vaccine effectiveness.

The vaccine genie will be hard to put back in the bottle. Time will tell.

Herpes Zoster (Shingles)

According to the CDC, herpes zoster, also known as shingles, is caused by reactivation of varicella-zoster virus (VZV), the same virus that causes varicella (chickenpox). After a person has varicella, the virus remains latent in the dorsal root ganglia (a clump of nerves that serves as a hub connecting the spinal cord or cranial nerves to regions of the body). VZV can reactivate later in a person's life and cause herpes zoster, a painful maculopapular and then vesicular rash.[12]

In about 70% of cases, the varicella virus remains dormant in the body, hiding out in nerve root ganglia. These ganglia can be anywhere along the spinal cord or the cranial nerves. Under certain conditions such as stress, immune suppression, or aging, the dormant herpes zoster virus can erupt as shingles. The rash of shingles typically follows the pattern of nerve distribution to the skin, hence the typical geographic shape.

Shingles Is More Than Just a Rash

The rate of serious complications from shingles is far greater than complications from chickenpox.

Long-term nerve pain called postherpetic neuralgia (PHN) is the most common complication of shingles, occurring in about 10-18% of people, and the risk and severity increases with age. The pain occurs where the shingles rash is located and can persist long after the rash subsides–months or even years. The pain is difficult to treat and can be quite debilitating, even interfering with daily life. There is no cure.

In rare instances, shingles can also lead to infection of the lungs, hearing problems, encephalitis, and even death.

Ocular Shingles

In around 9% of shingles cases, the eruption involves the eye. The symptoms can be severe and include blisters around the upper eyelid and forehead, burning or throbbing around the eye, eye redness, tearing, and blurry vision. The blisters and rash may resolve after a few weeks, but the eye pain and skin sensitivity can be permanent.

Shingles Does Not Mean Loss of Natural Immunity

As stated before, chickenpox infection confers lifelong natural immunity. A shingles breakout is not the same as the kind of reinfection that might occur with waning vaccine effectiveness. Rather, shingles signal a reactivation of the virus that has lain dormant in the body, often for decades.

Are We Seeing Other Trade-offs for Vaccination?

A significant trade-off may be in progress, and that is a decrease in cases of chickenpox but a rise in shingles cases . . . and the two may be connected.

A multi-year study funded by the CDC tracked the incidence of chickenpox cases in a region of California after introduction of the varicella vaccine.[13] A few years later, shingles surveillance (reporting and tracking cases) was added to the project.

As expected, there was a significant decline in chickenpox cases. Quite unexpectedly however, there was a large increase in shingles cases in adults aged 26-69 years, jumping nearly 30% in one year.

Medical costs of caring for shingles can be four to five times higher than caring for chickenpox.[14] The California study authors expressed concern that medical cost savings from large reductions in chickenpox will be more than offset by the costs driven by increased shingles cases.

Interestingly, one of the reasons the UK does not include chickenpox vaccination in the National Health Service vaccine schedule is due to lack of cost-effectiveness.

A larger study done by the CDC several years later had similar findings to the California results.[15] The CDC reported that the incidence of shingles in adults ages thirty to sixty years old in particular has been climbing since 2008, while the rate in older adults has been stable since that time.

The exact reason for this increase is unknown, but there is evidence that the prevalence of natural chickenpox in the community may help prevent shingles in adulthood. One study performed in the UK, where the varicella vaccine is not a regularly administered childhood vaccine, showed that adults exposed to chickenpox as a result of living with children decreased the likelihood of shingles by 30% over twenty years.[16]

> Cell-mediated immunity is a key mechanism whereby the immune system suppresses the reemergence of the varicella zoster virus that causes shingles.

It is thought that re-exposure to chickenpox during adulthood helps to boost cell-mediated immunity in the previously infected.[17] In other words, periodic exposure to chickenpox in adulthood helps to maintain cellular immunity, a key mechanism by which the varicella-zoster virus is suppressed.

Despite this evidence, the CDC denies there is any correlation between chickenpox vaccination and the rising incidence of shingles.

The Downside of Herd Immunity

The UK study calls into question whether the CDC has adequately considered longer-term risk from vaccination.

Human immune systems have been contending with highly infectious viruses for millennia. The introduction of vaccines inevitably distorts the finely tuned balance of immune system protection.

After the introduction of mass varicella vaccination in 1995, herd immunity was rapidly attained, and the chickenpox virus was no longer in wide circulation. This meant that those who had been infected prior to introduction of the vaccine and harbored the virus in their nervous system were no longer getting re-exposed to the virus.

The loss of ongoing immune system stimulation from viral re-exposure may have led to a jump in shingles cases in the previously infected as they aged. People currently in their mid-thirties and up would most likely have been infected prior to roll-out of the vaccine. Ironically, herd immunity may have removed the one essential ingredient for ongoing immune system stimulation necessary to prevent reactivation of the varicella-zoster virus.

The apparent lack of impact of herd immunity on those 60+ may simply be due to the fact that this group already has a much higher incidence of shingles and that the loss of environmental exposure to the virus has had less effect.

Vaccine Does Not Significantly Impact Developing Childhood Immune, Cardiovascular, Neurological, Hematological, Hormonal, or Musculoskeletal Systems—B

Serious reactions to the vaccine are rare but can include pneumonia, infection of the brain and/or spinal cord covering, or seizures that are often associated with fever. Longer-term risks include waning immunity, which can result in more serious infection as an adult.

Herd immunity to chickenpox may increase the chance of shingles in adults, which has a much higher rate of serious side effects than from an initial chickenpox infection.

Increasing incidence of shingles has necessitated shingles vaccination. Hence, another vaccine is necessary to address conditions that may be exacerbated by vaccination in the first place.

Vaccine Creates Lifelong Immunity—C

Thus far, immunity has only been established for ten years.

Vaccine Important to Achieve Herd Immunity—B

The vaccine is considered important to achieve herd immunity. However, as noted above, herd immunity due to vaccination may have a paradoxical effect on the incidence of shingles in adults over sixty.

Overall Grade—B

High-risk children and adults may benefit from vaccination. Healthy children may have more potential risk than benefit from immunization against chickenpox when the absolute risk reduction is taken into account. Several Western nations do not offer the vaccine, and others delay initial vaccination until after ten years of age.

Postponing the first vaccination until elementary school seems a reasonable trade-off for healthy children who have not been infected or who have not developed antibodies by that age. The Varicella-Zoster Virus (VZV) titer test, also known as the VZV antibody or Chickenpox test, is readily available and does not even require a doctor's prescription. Results should help to guide the decision to vaccinate.

Women who are pregnant or who may become pregnant and are uncertain if they've had the vaccine or chickenpox should get the blood test to decide if they are immune.

The ultimate tradeoff between public benefits and the risks/costs of reinfection and shingles have yet to be determined. The assumption of great benefits compared to little risk from mass vaccination deserves reexamination.

CHAPTER 12

Haemophilus influenzae b Vaccine (Hib)

Haemophilus influenzae is a bacterial disease that is transmitted person-to-person by respiratory droplets. It is not highly contagious, but exposure under crowded conditions (e.g., household, childcare, or institutional setting) can lead to outbreaks.[1] Other risk factors include age (under two years), Native American ethnicity, chronic diseases, and immune deficiency. Breastfed infants may be protected by maternal antibodies for up to six months.[2]

Pre-vaccine, the disease caused only about 20,000 infections a year in the US; this has dropped by 99% since introduction of the vaccine in 1993.[3] Some infections can invade the bloodstream, resulting in potentially life-threatening disorders such as meningitis, epiglottitis, and pneumonia.[4] Treatment consists of hospitalization, antibiotics, and supportive care.

Criteria	Grade
Children are at high risk of severe illness or death from disease	A
Vaccine prevents infection and replication	C
Vaccine prevents transmission to others	B
Vaccine is approved for use by the FDA	A
Vaccine safety and efficacy supported by randomized, controlled, clinical trials	D
Vaccine does not significantly impact developing childhood immune, cardiovascular, neurological, hematological, hormonal, or musculoskeletal systems	B
Vaccine creates lifelong immunity	C
Vaccine important to achieve herd immunity	A
Overall Grade	**B**

Vaccine Schedule

The CDC recommends routine administration of a conjugate Hib vaccine series beginning at age two months.

Specifically, infants two to six months old receive either:

1. A three-dose series of ActHIB®, Hiberix®, Pentacel®, or Vaxelis®
2. A two-dose series of PedvaxHIB®

Next, the CDC recommends a booster dose of any licensed conjugate Hib vaccine at age twelve through fifteen months.[5]

Vaccines Offered

The FDA categorizes the Hib vaccine as a polysaccharide conjugate.[6] Hib conjugate vaccines are prepared by combining the H. influenzae capsular outer shell with protein extractions from diphtheria, meningococcal, or tetanus bacteria (a different one for each of the three Hib conjugate vaccines).

There are five types of Haemophilus influenzae type b (Hib) vaccines authorized for use in the United States. Of these, three are monovalent conjugate vaccines, and two are combination vaccines.

The conjugation is necessary because the H. influenza capsule does not elicit an adequate immune response on its own and needs foreign proteins to boost the immune reaction. These vaccine conjugates do not take the place of the regular vaccines for diphtheria, tetanus, or meningococcus that children and adults should receive.

Monovalent Conjugate Hib Vaccines

Vaccine	**Excipients**[7]
ActHIB® (PRP-T)	*None*
Hiberix® (PRP-T)	formaldehyde, sodium chloride, lactose
PedvaxHIB® (PRP-OMB)	amorphous aluminum hydroxyphosphate sulfate, sodium chloride

Combination Vaccines (that contain Hib vaccine)

Vaccine	**Excipients**[8]
Pentacel®	aluminum phosphate, polysorbate 80, sucrose, formaldehyde, glutaraldehyde, bovine serum albumin, 2-phenoxyethanol, neomycin, polymyxin B sulfate
Vaxeli®	polysorbate 80, formaldehyde, glutaraldehyde, bovine serum albumin, neomycin, streptomycin sulfate, polymyxin B sulfate, ammonium thiocyanate, yeast protein, aluminum

Contraindications include hypersensitivity to any component of the vaccine or the diluent.[9]

Children Are at High Risk of Severe Illness or Death from Disease—A

H. influenza infection was not common prior to the introduction of vaccines in 1993, with about 20,000 cases per year. Post-vaccine, that number has dropped significantly. Despite the small number of cases, infections may result in life-threatening, invasive disease.

Vaccine Prevents Infection and Replication—C

H. influenza is not easily transmitted between individuals. Most infections colonize the nasopharynx and cause no clinical disease. Although the number of infections has declined markedly since introduction of the vaccine, the rate of invasive H. influenzae infections paradoxically increased from 1.23 per 100,000 population in 1997 to 2.08 per 100,000 population in 2018. Researchers report that the increased incidence of invasive disease is being driven by strains (serotype a & non-typeable) not covered by the vaccine, suggesting that other strains are taking the place of H. Influenza b.[10]

Vaccine Prevents Transmission to Others—B

H. influenza is not easily transmitted. Hib only covers the b strain, and does not prevent the transmission of other H. influenza strains a through f that are growing in prevalence. However, the marked decline in cases to date after introduction of the vaccine suggests some interruption of both replication and transmission.

Vaccine Is Approved for Use by the FDA—A

The vaccine is approved for use by the FDA.

Vaccine Safety and Efficacy Supported by Randomized, Controlled, Clinical Trials—D

Safety

Adverse events following vaccination include:

- Immune system disorders: Anaphylaxis, other allergic/hypersensitivity reactions (including urticaria, angioedema)
- Nervous system disorders: Convulsions, Guillain-Barre'
- General disorders and administration site conditions: Extensive limb swelling, peripheral edema, pruritus, rash (including generalized rash)

None of the vaccines have been evaluated for their carcinogenic or mutagenic potential or impairment of male fertility.

Efficacy

None of the approved Hib vaccines has been subjected to a randomized, controlled clinical trial. All have had immunogenic studies only, where antibody levels are measured post-vaccination. According to the CDC, vaccine protective efficacy based on immunogenic results is between 93% and 100%.[11]

All three vaccines have only been tested against other Hib vaccines, Hib vaccines combined with other vaccines, or other vaccines such as DTP or OPV as controls. Only one of the three vaccines has been compared with a placebo in one of its immunogenicity trials; the contents of that placebo have not been published.[12]

As a result, Relative Risk Reduction and Absolute Risk Reduction cannot be calculated.

Vaccine Does Not Significantly Impact Developing Childhood Immune, Cardiovascular, Neurological, Hematological, Hormonal, or Musculoskeletal Systems—B

Information is lacking about the effect of the vaccine on developing systems in young children, although reported systemic effects such as seizures and Guillain-Barré syndrome implicate the vaccine as a potential cause of nervous system inflammation.

Vaccine Creates Lifelong Immunity—C

The duration of immunity is at least several years, but lifelong immunity has not been established. Suppression of the b strain by Hib and backfilling by other known strains suggests immunity to H. influenza may wane over time.

Vaccine Important for Herd Immunity—A

Hib has been established as an important contributor to herd immunity. It remains to be seen if backfilling strains will diminish its role in herd immunity over time.

Overall Grade—B

The disease is rare, but the risks of severe illness if infected are high.

CHAPTER 13

Hepatitis A Vaccine (HepA)

The Most Effective Vaccine . . . That Children Don't Need

Hepatitis A (HepA) is an extremely contagious liver infection. Transmission occurs when the virus is ingested, even in microscopic amounts, via close contact with an infected person or through contaminated food. Most infected children are asymptomatic or have mild illness; however, they can pass the disease to family members or caregivers who don't have immunity.[1]

Older persons who contract hepatitis A experience symptoms, which can be quite severe, for two to six months.[2] Unlike Hepatitis B, which can result in becoming a chronic carrier, infection with hepatitis A provides lifelong immunity.

In 1996, the CDC recommended HepA vaccination for certain populations, including children living in communities at high risk for contracting the disease. Ten years later, they updated their recommendation to include routine vaccination of all children beginning at twelve months. Symptoms typically appear two to seven weeks post-transmission and can include yellow skin and eyes, stomach and joint pain, fever, vomiting, and fatigue. There are no medications available to treat hepatitis A, so physicians often recommend rest, adequate nutrition, and fluids.[3]

Criteria	Grade
Children are at high risk of severe illness or death from disease	F
Vaccine prevents infection and replication	A
Vaccine prevents transmission to others	A
Vaccine is approved for use by the FDA	A
Vaccine safety and efficacy supported by randomized, controlled, clinical trials	D
Vaccine does not significantly impact developing childhood immune, cardiovascular, neurological, hematological, hormonal, or musculoskeletal systems	D

(Continued on next page)

Criteria	Grade
Vaccine creates lifelong immunity	B
Vaccine important to reach herd immunity	B
Overall Grade	**B**

Vaccine Schedule

The CDC recommends that all children receive two doses of the hepatitis A vaccine. The first dose is administered between 12-23 months and the second at least six months later. If a child is not vaccinated within that time frame, the CDC maintains that vaccination should be administered to children 2–18 years old as well.[4]

Vaccines Offered

There are two single-antigen, inactivated virus HepA vaccines licensed for use in children in the United States.

Vaccine	Excipients
Havrix®	MRC-5 cellular proteins, formalin, aluminum hydroxide, amino acid supplement, phosphate-buffered saline solution, polysorbate 20, neomycin sulfate, aminoglycoside antibiotic
Vaqta®	amorphous aluminum hydroxyphosphate sulfate, non-viral protein, DNA, bovine albumin, formaldehyde, neomycin, sodium borate, sodium chloride, other process chemical residuals

These vaccines can be administered on their own or concurrently with other vaccines.[5]

Contraindications include an allergic reaction after a previous dose of hepatitis A vaccine and any severe, life-threatening allergies.[6]

Children Are at High Risk of Severe Illness or Death from Disease—F

The vast majority of children who contract hepatitis A are either asymptomatic or experience mild illness. Infection gives lifelong immunity.

Vaccine Prevents Infection, Replication, and Transmission—A

Hepatitis A vaccines are highly effective at preventing infection, replication, and transmission to other children based on Relative Risk Reduction measures. Unfortunately, since the introduction of the vaccines in 1999, the burden of disease has shifted to persons older than twenty years of age.[7]

According to the CDC,

This has resulted in the average age of hepatitis A-related hospitalizations and deaths increasing, and the proportion of persons hospitalized is more likely to have liver diseases and other comorbid medical conditions.[8]

Vaccine Is Approved for Use by the FDA—A

Vaccine Safety and Efficacy Supported by Randomized, Controlled, Clinical Trials—D

Safety

Hepatitis A vaccines were not subjected to randomized, controlled clinical trials. Clinical trials found a high incidence of irritability, drowsiness, and loss of appetite. The vaccines were tested against other hepatitis vaccines, excipients only, or no controls. The vaccines were not tested for carcinogenesis, mutagenesis, or impact on fertility.[9]

Post-marketing studies of adverse events found evidence for thrombocytopenia (low platelet count), Guillain-Barré syndrome, encephalitis, and cerebellar ataxia.[10]

Excipients include aluminum phosphate and aluminum hydroxide. While aluminum compounds can be an effective adjuvant, they are also known neurotoxins.[11] The metal is well-absorbed when injected, can be especially harmful to the brain and nerves, and has been implicated in diseases such as Alzheimer's, autism, and multiple sclerosis. Aluminum has also been implicated in triggering autoimmune disorders. See Chapter 2, First, Do No Harm for a discussion of aluminum toxicity.

Effectiveness

The estimated Relative Risk Reduction (RRR) for the vaccine was between 84% and 94%. The Absolute Risk Reduction (ARR) was roughly 0.2% for Havrix® based on data provided in the package inserts. Vaqta® was only tested for antibody response to hepatitis A and not subjected to clinical trials.[12] Therefore, the RRR and ARR for Vaqta® are not known.

Vaccine Does Not Significantly Impact Developing Childhood Immune, Cardiovascular, Neurological, Hematological, Hormonal, or Musculoskeletal Systems—D

Excipients aluminum phosphate and aluminum hydroxide are known neurotoxins.[13] The metal is especially harmful to the brain and nerves and has been implicated in diseases such as Alzheimer's, autism, and multiple sclerosis.[14,15,16]

Vaccine Creates Lifelong Immunity—B

The duration of immunity is unknown in children, but anti-hepatitis A antibodies have been detected in vaccinated adults for twenty years or more.[17] The concern about widespread vaccination in children is reflected in the increasing incidence of hepatitis A in persons twenty years and older. It is unclear whether this represents a waning of immunity or some other phenomenon.

Vaccine Important to Reach Herd Immunity—B

The large decline in the prevalence of hepatitis A among children after the introduction of the vaccine is likely due to an effect on herd immunity. However, since most children were infected before the vaccine and gained lifelong immunity, it appears the burden of herd immunity has now been shifted to vaccination. The rising incidence of infection in persons twenty years of age and older raises concerns about the long-term benefits of widespread childhood vaccination on public health.

Overall Grade—B

Hepatitis A vaccine may just be the most effective vaccine children do not need. Improvements in sanitation, personal hygiene, and public health have reduced the need to protect children from hepatitis A via vaccination. It is certainly preferable that children get infected during early childhood when they are asymptomatic or experience mild disease and thereby obtain lifelong immunity. In contrast, shifting the burden of disease to older years when the infection can have devastating consequences appears to be the price of widespread childhood vaccination.

This vaccine should be reconsidered for use on high-risk populations only.

CHAPTER 14

Inactivated Poliovirus Vaccine (IPV)

Polio (poliovirus) is a highly contagious infectious disease caused by a virus. Transmission occurs via droplets from a sneeze or cough or by contact with contaminated food, water, or the feces of an infected person. Polio can live in the intestines for several weeks and even asymptomatic carriers can pass the virus to others.[1] For the most part, polio affects children, but anyone who hasn't been vaccinated runs the risk of contracting the disease.[2]

In 1998, around 350,000 cases of polio were present throughout 125 countries. That number dropped substantially since the vaccine was introduced, and in 2022 there were only 30 cases across three countries.[3] Approximately 25% of people with poliovirus infection will experience flu-like symptoms. 1-5% will develop meningitis, and .5% will develop paralysis.[4] Post-polio Syndrome can occur decades after the initial infection and affects 25-40% of polio survivors.[5] Polio is not a curable disease, so treatments like antispasmodic drugs, heat, and physical therapy are used to alleviate symptoms and improve mobility.[6]

Criteria	Grade
Children are at high risk of severe illness or death from disease	B
Vaccine prevents infection and replication	B
Vaccine prevents transmission to others	C
Vaccine is approved for use by the FDA	A
Vaccine safety and efficacy supported by randomized, controlled, clinical trials	C
Vaccine does not significantly impact developing childhood immune, cardiovascular, neurological, hematological, hormonal, or musculoskeletal systems	B
Vaccine creates lifelong immunity	C
Vaccine important for herd immunity	B
Overall Grade	**B**

Vaccine Schedule

The CDC recommends that all children receive four doses of the inactivated polio vaccine. Doses are administered at two, four, and six to eighteen months, with a final dose administered between four to six years old.

Vaccines Offered

Two types of single-antigen inactivated polio vaccine products are licensed in the United States: IPOL® and POLIOVAX®.[7] Currently, IPOL is the only polio vaccine being used as POLIOVAX® was discontinued in 1991.[8]

Vaccine	Excipients[9]
IPOL®	calf bovine serum albumin, 2-phenoxyethanol, formaldehyde, neomycin, streptomycin, polymyxin B, M-199 medium

IPOL can be administered on its own, and it is also part of several combination vaccines, including:

Vaccine	Excipients[10]
Pentacel® (DTaP-IPV/Hib)	aluminum phosphate, polysorbate 80, sucrose, formaldehyde, glutaraldehyde, bovine serum albumin, 2-phenoxyethanol, neomycin, polymyxin B sulfate
Pediarix® (DTaP-IPV-HepB)	formaldehyde, aluminum hydroxide, aluminum phosphate, sodium chloride, polysorbate 80 (Tween 80), neomycin sulfate, polymyxin B, yeast protein
Kinrix® (DTaP-IPV)	formaldehyde, aluminum hydroxide, sodium chloride, polysorbate 80 (Tween 80), neomycin sulfate, polymyxin B
VAXELIS® (DTaP-IPV-Hib-HepB)	polysorbate 80, formaldehyde, glutaraldehyde, bovine serum albumin, neomycin, streptomycin sulfate, polymyxin B sulfate, ammonium thiocyanate, yeast protein, aluminum
Quadracel® (DTaP-IPV)	polysorbate 80, formaldehyde, glutaraldehyde, bovine serum albumin, neomycin, streptomycin sulfate, polymyxin B sulfate, ammonium thiocyanate, yeast protein, aluminum

Contraindications include hypersensitivity and anaphylactic reactions. Specifically, those who have experienced severe allergic reactions after a previous dose of inactivated polio vaccine (IPV) or after taking streptomycin, polymyxin B, or neomycin should not receive IPV.[11]

Children Are at High Risk of Severe Illness or Death from Disease—B

Over 90% of polio cases are asymptomatic and serious infections including acute flaccid paralysis are rare. More typically, symptoms resemble a minor illness. Clean drinking water, wastewater treatment, pasteurized foods, sanitary food supply chains, and proper personal and community sanitation have markedly diminished the risk of polio in developed nations.

Vaccine Prevents Infection and Replication—B

IPV induces production of an antibody (IgA) in the throat and intestines that reduces, but does not eliminate, polio virus excretion. Consequently, the polio virus is able to replicate in the intestines, but its ability to cause severe illness and paralysis (infection) is diminished by vaccination.

The oral polio vaccine (OPV), no longer available in this country, was more effective at preventing replication as well as infection. OPV, which had attenuated but not killed virus, was withdrawn in the US in 2000 due to OPV occasionally reverting to an active virus in the body, triggering polio infection.

Vaccine Prevents Transmission to Others—C

IPV does not prevent transmission, but the virus may be weakened as it passes through the intestine. Vaccinated children can still pass the virus to others through fecal transmission, but those who pick up the virus are less likely to contract the disease.

Vaccine Is Approved for Use by the FDA—A

The vaccine is approved by the FDA.

Vaccine Safety and Efficacy Supported by Randomized, Controlled, Clinical Trials—C

There are no randomized, placebo-controlled clinical trials proving the safety or efficacy of IPV. The vaccine was never tested for carcinogenesis, mutagenesis, or impact on fertility.

Post-marketing surveillance (monitoring the vaccine after approval) of IPV vaccine adverse events include swollen lymph glands, agitation, acute allergic reactions including anaphylaxis, sore joints and muscles, rash, skin eruptions, seizures, headache, abnormal sensations in the extremities, sleepiness, and loss of consciousness. Although no causal relationship has been established, deaths have occurred after vaccination of infants with IPV.[12]

Unlike oral polio vaccines, there is no evidence that IPV can transmit polio via vaccination.

People who are allergic to any of the vaccine's excipients, such as streptomycin, polymyxin B, and neomycin, may experience an allergic reaction including anaphylaxis.

Two doses of IPV are 90% effective or more against paralytic polio; three doses are 99-100% effective. The duration of IPV is unknown (see Lifelong Immunity section below).

Vaccine Does Not Significantly Impact Developing Childhood Immune, Cardiovascular, Neurological, Hematological, Hormonal, or Musculoskeletal Systems—B

The impact of IPV on a child's developing organ systems is difficult to ascertain as it is often given in combination with other vaccines. However, all inactivated viral vaccines contain killed virus plus excipients, and both are known to stimulate an inflammatory response. The effect of inflammation on immature immune, neurological, and other systems is poorly understood and harm cannot be excluded.

Vaccine Creates Lifelong Immunity—C

Killed virus vaccines are not as effective as attenuated, live virus vaccines. The duration of immunity is not known for children who receive a full IPV series, as IPV is the only type of polio vaccine that has been given in the US since 2000. Most are likely protected for many years. A 2009–2010 national survey showed that a high percentage of children and adults had protective antibodies even decades later.[13]

However, surveyed immunized adults had exposure to live, attenuated oral polio vaccine which is known to elicit more lasting immunity than IPV. Thus, the survey was limited in its ability to predict the duration of immunity for children who exclusively receive IPV. As the absolute duration of effectiveness is unknown, adults who are at higher risk of exposure (e.g. travel to countries where polio is endemic) should receive one lifetime IPV booster.

Vaccine Important for Herd Immunity—B

As noted above, the vaccine does not prevent replication or transmission. However, polio virus excreted by vaccinated individuals may be less infective. There is some evidence that herd immunity can be maintained in a population vaccinated only with IPV.[14] However, it is difficult to separate out other factors in developed nations that may be contributing to suppression of outbreaks.

Overall Grade—B

IPV is effective at preventing serious infection and building herd immunity. The currently approved killed virus vaccine is not as effective as the attenuated, live vaccine no longer available in the US, and viral shedding does occur. IPOL® does not contain aluminum excipients in contrast to all the combination vaccines that include IPV.

CHAPTER 15

Pneumococcal Conjugate Vaccine (PCV)

Pneumococcal disease is caused by the bacterium Streptococcus pneumoniae.[1] S. pneumoniae can infect children's lungs, middle ears, sinuses, lining of the brain and spinal cord, joints, bones, and blood. Pneumococcal pneumonia can be contagious and is transmitted through airborne respiratory droplets dispersed when an infected person coughs, sneezes, or talks. It is also possible, though less common, to contract pneumonia from touching a contaminated object or surface and then touching the nose or mouth.[2]

Children under five (especially premature infants), elderly, smokers, and those with chronic illness have an increased risk of contracting pneumonia[3] as do children of certain racial and ethnic groups including Alaskan Native, African American, and certain American Indian people.[4]

Symptoms of pneumonia include chest pain, cough, fever/chills, rapid breathing, and difficulty breathing. Complications include empyema, pericarditis, and endobronchial obstruction; this illness is fatal for one out of every twenty affected people, most of whom fall into a high-risk group.[5] Antibiotics are typically prescribed to treat pneumonia, and although some pneumococcal bacteria have become resistant, the CDC notes that the number of antibiotic-resistant pneumococcal infections has decreased due to the implementation of pneumococcal conjugate vaccination.[6]

The CDC began surveillance on pneumococcal disease in 1998; they recommended all children receive the pneumonia vaccine for the first time in 2000. Between 1998 and 2021, pneumonia cases in children under five years decreased by 95% overall.[7]

Criteria	Grade
Children are at high risk of severe illness or death from disease	C
Vaccine prevents infection and replication	C
Vaccine prevents transmission to others	B

Criteria	Grade
Vaccine is approved for use by the FDA	A
Vaccine safety and efficacy supported by randomized, controlled, clinical trials	C
Vaccine does not significantly impact developing childhood immune, cardiovascular, neurological, hematological, hormonal, or musculoskeletal systems	C
Vaccine creates lifelong immunity	D
Vaccine important to achieve herd immunity	B
Overall Grade	C

Vaccine Schedule

The CDC recommends pneumococcal vaccination for all children younger than 5. Most children receive four doses at two, four, six, and twelve to fifteen months. Children 2–18 years old with certain health conditions like HIV and sickle cell disease are at increased risk and may need additional doses.[8]

Vaccines Offered

The CDC recommends two kinds of pneumococcal vaccines:

- Pneumococcal conjugate vaccines (PCVs)
- PCVs are made by combining small pieces of pneumococcal bacteria outer shells with proteins from other bacteria.

Vaccine	Excipients[9]
PCV15 (Vaxneuvance®)	aluminum as aluminum phosphate
PCV20 (Prevnar 20®)	aluminum as aluminum phosphate

- Pneumococcal polysaccharide vaccine (PPSV23)
- PPSV23 consists of small pieces of pneumococcal bacteria outer shells.

Vaccine	Excipients[10]
PPSV23 (Pneumovax23®)	isotonic saline solution, phenol (no aluminum)

According to the CDC, the above vaccines can be administered at the same time as other routine childhood vaccinations except for Menactra®, a meningococcal conjugate vaccine.[11] PCV15 and PCV20 are approved for children under five years of age, and as young as six weeks. PPSV23 is restricted to children two years or older who are at increased risk of pneumococcal disease.

Contraindications for PCVs include previous severe allergic reaction after any type of PCV vaccine or any vaccine containing diphtheria toxoid (for example, DTaP). People should not receive the PPSV23 vaccine in cases of previous severe allergic reaction to the same. Anyone with a severe, life-threatening allergy to any excipient of these vaccines should not get that vaccine.[12]

Children Are at High Risk of Severe Illness or Death from Disease—C

Children are generally not at high risk from pneumonia unless they fall into certain risk groups such as premature birth, sickle cell disease, diabetes, asthma, bronchopulmonary dysplasia, immune suppression, and cystic fibrosis.

Vaccine Prevents Infection and Replication—C

None of the approved vaccines has been directly shown to prevent infection or replication, except for Prevnar20®, which was effective for most symptoms but showed weak efficacy (57%) against acute otitis media (severe ear infection) caused by pneumococcal disease.

The often cited 97–100% efficacy of PCV at pneumonia prevention was not tested in any of the approved vaccines (PCV15, PCV20, PPSV23). Instead, all three underwent antibody tests that measure response to the strains covered by the vaccine, not actual clinical trials in children.

Antibody studies are often used as a proxy for clinical trials as they are much easier to do and theoretically translated to clinical effectiveness. Unfortunately, antibody studies do not always correlate with clinical outcomes and should not be used as substitutes for actual disease prevention or mitigation.[13]

The manufacturer reasoned, and the FDA accepted, that results from earlier versions of the PCV vaccines would automatically apply to the newer vaccines since they are "manufactured similarly."[14] That assumption remains open to debate. A clinical study performed in Finland found PCV to be only 44% effective at preventing acute otitis media due to pneumococcal strains covered by the vaccine.

Not only was the vaccine marginally effective, but there was an increase in strains not covered by the vaccine, suggesting that PCV vaccinated children may be at increased risk of acute otitis media due to uncovered strains.[15]

Vaccine Prevents Transmission to Others—B

PCVs appear to prevent transmission of strains covered by the vaccine, but do not prevent infection or transmission of non-covered pneumococcal strains.

Vaccine Is Approved for Use by the FDA—A

PCV15, PCV20, and PPSV23 are all FDA approved for use in children as young as six weeks, except for PPSV23, which is restricted to children aged two or older who are considered high-risk.

Vaccine Safety and Efficacy Supported by Randomized, Controlled, Clinical Trials—C

Safety

Control groups are critical when it comes to assessing safety. None of the PCVs were compared with true placebos; instead, they were all compared with either earlier versions (meaning fewer strains covered) or with other pediatric vaccines such as meningococcal vaccine. As a result, adverse events in the "control" group are generally much higher than would be found in a placebo-controlled group. A greater rate of adverse events in the control group serves to mask or normalize the rate of adverse events found in the test group.

Post-Marketing Surveillance

Post-approval, manufacturers must collect information about adverse events that are potentially caused by their vaccines. The information is usually a mix of active and passive data collection, so rates of adverse events per number of doses given aren't always available.

Combined post-marketing data for Prevnar 10®, Prevnar 15®, PNEUMOVAX 23® are as follows:[16]

- General disorders and local reactions
  - Cellulitis, malaise, fever, (>102°F), drowsiness: >40% in individuals less than two years old
  - Irritability: >60% in individuals less than two years old
  - Warmth at the injection site, decreased limb mobility, peripheral edema in the injected extremity, injection-site necrosis
- Cardiac disorders
  - Cyanosis (pediatric populations only)
- Digestive System
  - Nausea
  - Vomiting
- Hematologic/Lymphatic
  - Lymphadenitis, lymphadenopathy, thrombocytopenia in patients with stabilized idiopathic thrombocytopenic purpura
  - Hemolytic anemia (in patients who have had other hematologic disorders)
  - Leukocytosis
- Hypersensitivity
  - Anaphylactoid reactions, serum Sickness, angioneurotic edema
- Musculoskeletal System
  - Arthralgia
  - Arthritis
- Nervous System

    - Hypotonia
    - Paresthesia
    - Radiculoneuropathy
    - Guillain-Barré syndrome
    - Febrile convulsion
- Respiratory
    - Apnea
- Skin
    - Rash
    - Urticaria
    - Cellulitis-like reactions
    - Erythema multiforme
- Vascular
    - Pallor
- Under Investigation
    - Increased serum C-reactive protein (biological marker of inflammation)

None of the PCVs have been evaluated for the potential to cause carcinogenicity, genotoxicity, or impairment of male fertility.

Efficacy

See discussion under Vaccine Prevents Infection and Replication (p. 128) for vaccine efficacy.

Vaccine Does Not Significantly Impact Developing Childhood Immune, Cardiovascular, Neurological, Hematological, Hormonal, or Musculoskeletal Systems—C

Post-marketing surveillance indicates a moderate to high risk of long-term complications from PCVs. In addition, none of the PCVs have been evaluated for the potential to cause carcinogenicity, genotoxicity, or impairment of male fertility. Therefore, it is not possible to ensure that PCVs will have no impact on these systems.

Vaccine Creates Lifelong Immunity—D

PCVs do not result in lifelong immunity. Covered strains are replaced by uncovered strains over time, rendering lifelong immunity improbable. Moreover, individuals may become at high risk for infection as they age due to the onset of chronic illnesses or simply the aging process.

Vaccine Important to Achieve Herd Immunity—B

There is partial herd protection for covered strains. An earlier version of the vaccine, PCV7, resulted in significant reductions in pneumonia cases caused by the seven strains, particularly among older children and adults.[17] However, the jump from PCV7 to PCV13 was not accompanied by as much improvement in herd immunity. There is evidence that expansion of the number of pneumococcal strains covered by a vaccine has led to type replacement (backfilling) by non-vaccine strains.[18] Repeated expansion of the number of covered strains (now 23) may do little to improve herd immunity.

Overall Grade—C

The lack of clinical trials combined with the absence of placebo control groups undermines the CDC's confidence in the efficacy and safety of PCVs.

The evolution of PCVs shows a seemingly endless effort to expand the number of strains covered by the vaccines. Coverage started with 7 strains, then 10, 13, 15, 20, and now PPSV23. This strategy will inevitably lead to more backfilling by the remaining 70 or so strains and possibly more dangerous variants driven by PCV/ PPSV immune pressure.

CHAPTER 16

Rotavirus Vaccine

Rotavirus is a highly contagious disease that is transmitted via an infected person's stool. People with rotavirus can spread it prior to having symptoms and are most contagious at the onset of the illness and during the first three days post-recovery. Infants younger than three months of age have relatively low rates of rotavirus infection, probably because of passive maternal antibodies and possibly breastfeeding. The incidence of clinical illness is highest among children three to thirty-five months of age.

Transmission occurs when rotavirus particles enter the mouth through contaminated food or unwashed hands. The disease is easily spread among children and infants, who are most likely to be affected from January through June.[1]

Prior to the introduction of the rotavirus vaccine in 2006, this disease was the leading cause of severe diarrhea in infants and children in the US. Each year, the vaccine prevents 40,000 to 50,000 hospitalizations among this population, and the illness has decreased among unvaccinated adults and older children as well.[2] There isn't a specific medicine that treats the virus itself, but physicians often recommend medication aimed at easing symptoms which include vomiting, nausea, and diarrhea.[3]

Criteria	Grade
Children are at high risk of severe illness or death from disease	B
Vaccine prevents infection and replication	C
Vaccine prevents transmission to others	C
Vaccine is approved for use by the FDA	A
Vaccine safety and efficacy supported by randomized, controlled, clinical trials	C
Vaccine does not significantly impact developing childhood immune, cardiovascular, neurological, hematological, hormonal, or musculoskeletal systems	C
Vaccine creates lifelong immunity	C
Vaccine important to reach herd immunity	B
Overall Grade	**B**

Vaccine Schedule

The CDC recommends that all children receive the rotavirus vaccine. There are two vaccines licensed for infants in the US; one is given in two doses (two and four months), and the other is given in three doses (two, four, and six months). The first dose is given before fifteen weeks of age and the second before eight months. The rotavirus vaccine is administered via oral drops.[4]

Vaccines Offered

Vaccines	Excipients[5]
RotaTeq® (RV5): 3 doses at ages 2 months, 4 months, and 6 months	sucrose, sodium citrate, sodium phosphate monobasic monohydrate, sodium hydroxide, polysorbate 80, cell culture media, fetal bovine serum
Rotarix® (RV1): 2 doses at ages 2 months and 4 months	dextran, Dulbecco's Modified Eagle Medium (sodium chloride, potassium chloride, magnesium sulfate, ferric (III) nitrate, sodium phosphate, sodium pyruvate, D-glucose, concentrated vitamin solution, L-cystine, L-tyrosine, amino acids, L-glutamine, calcium chloride, sodium hydrogenocarbonate, and phenol red), sorbitol, sucrose, calcium carbonate, sterile water, xanthan [Porcine circovirus type 1 (PCV1) is present in Rotarix. PCV-1 is not known to cause disease in humans.]

According to the CDC, rotavirus vaccine can be administered at the same time as the DTaP vaccine, Hib vaccine, polio vaccine, hepatitis B vaccine, and pneumococcal conjugate vaccine.[6]

Contraindications include:[7]

- Severe allergic reaction to a previous dose of rotavirus vaccine
- Severe allergy to any component of rotavirus vaccine
- Severe combined immunodeficiency (SCID)
- Previous episode of intussusception (blockage from intestine telescoping into itself)

Children Are at High Risk of Severe Illness or Death from Disease—B

Rotavirus is extremely common in children, accounting for 5-10% of all cases of childhood gastroenteritis. According to the CDC, by age six, nearly every child will have an episode of rotavirus gastroenteritis, one in five will visit a clinic, one in 60 will be hospitalized, and approximately one in 293 will die.[8]

One study puts the estimated cumulative incidence by age five (the likelihood of hospital admission from a case of rotavirus over the course of five years) at a slightly lower rate of one rotavirus hospitalization per 108 children in the Medicaid population and one per 144 children in the non-Medicaid population.[9]

Watery diarrhea can rapidly lead to dehydration in children, especially in children under twelve months. Most children respond promptly to proper supportive care and rehydration.

Vaccine Prevents Infection and Replication—C

Two clinical trials found Rotarix® to have 85% protection against severe rotavirus gastroenteritis and 96% protection against hospitalization through two rotavirus seasons (December through June), both Relative Risk Reduction or RRR estimates.[10]

However, the Absolute Risk Reduction or ARR for any given child undergoing vaccination shows just 4.6% reduction in risk against severe rotavirus gastroenteritis across two seasons and only 0.9% reduction in risk against hospitalization (based on one season only).

In large clinical trials, RotaTeq® demonstrated 98% protection against severe rotavirus gastroenteritis (fever, vomiting, diarrhea, and changes in behavior), and 96% protection against hospitalization for rotavirus gastroenteritis.[11]

Again, analysis of Absolute Risk Reduction reveals far less impressive results. There was only a 2% reduction in risk of severe gastroenteritis following immunization and a 0.4% reduction in risk against hospitalization based on one season only.

Duration of protection wanes over the first few years, usually sufficient to protect against severe infection long enough to get past the most vulnerable years.

According to a 2019 study of hospital discharges, hospitalizations for rotavirus gastroenteritis among children ages four and under decreased by 86% between 2000 and 2013.[12]

Vaccine Prevents Transmission to Others—C

It is unclear from available data if RV prevents transmission or shedding of a weakened virus. However, the vaccine's live, attenuated virus can infect others post-vaccination.[13] Therefore caution is advised when considering whether the vaccine should be given to individuals with close contacts who may have depressed immune function from illness, cancer, therapies, or genetic immune deficiency.

Vaccine is Approved for Use by the FDA—A

The vaccine is approved for use by the FDA.

Vaccine Safety and Efficacy Supported by Randomized, Controlled, Clinical Trials—C

There are no randomized, placebo-controlled, clinical trials in support of either available vaccine. Safety and efficacy was determined by the vaccines being compared to only their excipients (i.e., the vaccine formula without the antigens). The vaccines have not been tested for carcinogenesis, mutagenicity, or for their impact on fertility.

According to the Rotarix® vaccine insert, adverse reactions within eight days of dose one and dose two were as follows:[14]

Adverse Reaction	Dose 1		Dose 2	
	ROTARIX® n = 3,284 %	Placebo n = 2,013 %	ROTARIX® n = 3,201 %	Placebo n = 1,973 %
Fussiness/irritability	52	52	42	42
Cough/runny nose	28	30	31	33
Fever	25	33	28	34
Loss of appetite	25	25	21	21
Vomiting	13	11	8	8
Diarrhea	4	3	3	3

Solicited adverse reactions within 8 days following doses 1 and 2 of ROTARIX or Placebo (Total Vaccinated Cohort = All vaccinated infants for whom safety data were available)

Aside from the high incidence of vaccine adverse events (which can be compounded by customary simultaneous administration of other vaccines), the minor differences with the placebo group are noteworthy. As noted, the vaccines were tested against themselves minus the rotavirus itself to form the placebo group.

The obvious implication is that the excipients are toxic and highly inflammatory, eliciting strong immune reactions. While a significant immune response is the intended purpose of excipients, it should not be forgotten that children receive heavy doses of these toxins with each and every vaccination.

Vaccine Does Not Significantly Impact Developing Childhood Immune, Cardiovascular, Neurological, Hematological, Hormonal, or Musculoskeletal Systems—C

Vaccine-related, severe adverse events include intussusception, recurrent intussusception (including death), hematochezia (passage of fresh blood per rectum), gastroenteritis with vaccine viral shedding in infants with SCID (Severe Combined Immune Deficiency Disorder), idiopathic thrombocytopenic purpura, and Kawasaki disease.[15] All have consequential residual implications for the health of a developing child.

As noted above, rotavirus vaccines contain significant amounts of excipients which cause strong inflammatory responses. The long-term implication of repeated exposure to such toxic excipients is unknown.

Vaccine Creates Lifelong Immunity—C

The duration of protection after a complete vaccination series has not been studied beyond the third season after vaccination.[16] Natural immunity is known to wane over time, as reinfections occur throughout life. However, infection provides effective defense against subsequent severe illness and the vaccines are likely to offer similar protection.[17]

Vaccine Important for Herd Immunity—B

There is considerable dispute about rotavirus vaccine impact on herd immunity. The vaccine likely does have an effect, possibly helping prevent severe disease and not infection, but it wanes over time. A meta-analysis of studies conducted to estimate herd protection in children twelve months old or less suggests a median herd effect on rotavirus gastroenteritis of just 22% across twelve study years.[18]

Overall Grade—B

Rotavirus vaccine has effectively reduced the incidence of severe rotavirus gastroenteritis and hospitalization for severe rotavirus gastroenteritis. However, the absolute risk reduction against these outcomes for any particular child is less impressive. Neither of the commercially available vaccines contain aluminum excipients.

PART FOUR

Special Considerations

CHAPTER 17

Why a Child Should Never, Ever Be Given an mRNA Vaccine

Let's start with some basics. Messenger RNA (mRNA) is found in every cell of the human body. Its job is to communicate messages, or code, from DNA in a cell's nucleus to the cell's protein manufacturing system. A cell's nucleus is unimaginably complex. It hosts around 25,000 segments of DNA, called genes, that are responsible for the genetic code that makes over 100,000 proteins essential for life.

Messenger RNA translates commands from the nucleus thousands of times a day, and after delivering its instructions, it's immediately broken down and recycled to form the next distinct mRNA genetic code as instructed by the cell's DNA inside the nucleus.

Before 2021, few people were familiar with the concept of an mRNA ***vaccine***. As it became better known during the COVID-19 pandemic, most thought of it as a step forward in the ongoing and inevitable march of science.

mRNA Vaccines

The idea of an mRNA vaccine comes from ancient foes: viruses like influenza, polio, and the common cold. These viruses cannot replicate on their own, so they have to find a host to supply all the ingredients they lack. Once viruses infect the body, they insidiously hijack a cell's protein-making machinery by inserting their own RNA or DNA into an unsuspecting cell, thereby creating billions of replicas of themselves.

As the newly born viruses burst forth from infected cells, the immune system attacks and destroys them–but usually not before the virus has been transmitted to other people.

mRNA vaccines work similarly. They insert their own genetic code into a cell and force it to produce not a whole virus but a single viral protein component. The goal is for the resulting proteins to sensitize the immune system to fight future attacks of a virus containing the same protein structure.

How Are mRNA Vaccines Different from Traditional Vaccines?

Whereas mRNA vaccines take over a cell to produce a single viral protein component, most other vaccines include weakened or killed viruses or bacteria. Some use recombinant technology to produce an antigen similar to the original virus to stimulate an immune response to the target pathogen.

> Recombinant viral vaccines are created by inserting genes from a virus into a host species (often yeast or bacteria) to produce a component of the virus that will serve as the antigen in the vaccine. In other words, the process uses the protein-making machinery of billions of yeast or bacterial cells to make the desired antigens used to produce a vaccine.

Prior to the mRNA vaccine, the FDA has never, in its entire history, authorized a vaccine that takes over a human cell's protein manufacturing process to produce a protein alien to the cell. This is a clear-cut alteration of normal, cellular gene expression. In other words, it is genetic manipulation, sometimes referred to as "gene therapy."

Strong objection has been made to calling mRNA vaccines gene therapy.[1] But Pfizer itself, one of two makers of mRNA COVID-19 vaccines, has said that mRNA technology is a good fit for gene editing, which means of course that the technology can be used to modify the expression of human DNA.[2]

Viruses have scores of antigens that the immune system recognizes in order to develop an effective and lasting immune response. Vaccines made up of weakened or killed viruses contain all or most of the original viral antigens. As a rule of thumb, the greater the number of antigens presented by a vaccine, the more complete and lasting the immune protection. However, an mRNA vaccine produces only a *single* protein antigen.

Why Natural Immunity Is Best

It has been known since the Athenian Plague of 430 BC that those who recover from an infection are protected if re-exposed to the disease.[3] Infection produces a robust and durable immunity in healthy children. The developing immune system gains exposure to all the antigens contained in a virus or other pathogen, allowing it to prepare for thousands of possible variants.

Both the innate (rapid response) immune system and the adaptive (long-term memory) immune system are activated by infection, and both are essential for locking in the capacity to fight off future infections.

On the other hand, immunity trained by a vaccine with a single or limited set of antigens, like the mRNA vaccine, may be caught flat-footed when variants of the original infection are encountered. Such was the case with SARS-CoV-2 when the original vaccine based on the Wuhan strain could only mount a limited and short-lived neutralizing immune response to Omicron variants.

modRNA

Most people, including many health-care providers, are unaware that COVID-19 vaccines don't actually contain mRNA but a modified version known as modRNA.

Unlike what the CDC told the public about how mRNA vaccines rapidly break down after injection, modRNA resists destruction by normal cellular enzymes. The persistence of modRNA inside of cells and continued production of foreign proteins can have significant, negative health consequences. More about this later—see **modRNA—It Was Never mRNA** below.

sa-mRNA

Researchers have developed another version of modified RNA, something called self-amplifying or sa-mRNA, that replicates its own modRNA once inside the cell. The first such self-copying RNA vaccine for COVID-19 won full approval in late 2023 in Japan.[4]

sa-mRNA continues production of antigens on its own using a person's own cells as a factory. In theory, a smaller dose of sa-mRNA would be needed to produce the equivalent amount of protein as higher doses of modRNA. However, even sa-mRNA is limited to a single antigen per vaccine, regardless of the amount.

sa-mRNA raises alarming questions. How does sa-mRNA know when to shut itself off? Does potential overproduction of a single antigen excessively focus the immune response (i.e., immune imprinting, as discussed below), thereby compromising immune response to future variants? Another concern is the potential for autoimmune disorders as a result of immune hyperstimulation.

Risks related to self-amplification may far outweigh any possible benefits.

modRNA Vaccines in the Pipeline

The pharmaceutical industry is enamored with mRNA or, more precisely, with the modRNA technology platform. The technology enables rapid prototyping of custom-tailored antigens that can be manufactured at vast scale through recombinant DNA technology.

> Recombinant DNA technology inserts a cloned (copied) gene into a bacterial cell to produce a desired gene product such as modRNA. The process is also used to make therapies such as insulin and growth hormone.

At least four mRNA flu vaccines have begun clinical trials, including those from Pfizer, Moderna, Sanofi, and the National Institute for Allergies and Infectious Diseases (NIAID).

For example, Moderna is developing modRNA vaccines for respiratory syncytial virus (RSV), Zika virus, HIV, Cytomegalovirus (CMV), COVID-19, influenza, and a combination COVID-19/Influenza vaccine.

In addition to influenza mRNA vaccines, Pfizer is working on a shingles vaccine and combination COVID-19/RSV and COVID-19/Influenza vaccines.

It's for Your "Convenience"

Combination vaccines are promoted for their convenience by minimizing the number of injections. However, they restrict choice when offered in combination and make full disclosure of benefits and risks of each separate vaccine more difficult. They are also a mechanism by which pharmaceutical companies can boost sales.

The industry is concerned about the steep drop off in sales following record profits from COVID-19 vaccines.[5] It seems public appetite for the relatively ineffective and potentially quite harmful vaccines has waned.

Vaccine manufacturers hope that by combining an established and generally accepted yearly shot like influenza vaccine with a vaccine whose sales are lagging, overall sales will pick back up.

As the president of Pfizer remarked recently during an investors call, he believes the convenience of offering combination vaccines will "unlock a significant potential by improving vaccination rates."[6]

Significant potential for whom?

Look for many new combination vaccines in the years to come to boost corporate bottom lines. Most of these products will use modRNA or sa-mRNA technologies and will be pitched to consumers as a convenience that unlocks "significant potential," but perhaps not human potential.

modRNA—It Was Never mRNA

As noted, mRNA is the highly efficient messenger system used by cells to produce proteins. mRNA is a single use system; once the coded protein is made, enzymes in the cell rapidly degrade the messenger RNA into its component parts, and it is then ready to be reassembled into a new strand of mRNA as needed.

Prompt breakdown of mRNA was the basis for the often-repeated phrase that mRNA in the COVID-19 vaccine rapidly disappears after it delivers instructions for the manufacture of the Spike protein.

modRNA Made to Be Stealthy and Durable

Just four molecules called nucleotides comprise all the genetic code carried by RNA. Variations in the length and sequence of these four molecules in mRNA set the code to determine which proteins are made.

However, BioNTech/Pfizer and Moderna modified the RNA code for the Spike protein by swapping out one of the naturally occurring nucleotides (uridine) and substituting a synthetic version called pseudouridine (officially *N*1-methylpseudouridine). Hence, modRNA.

Pfizer Confirms Use of modRNA

Although it takes some digging to find it amidst all the mRNA hype, the use of modRNA is confirmed by Pfizer on its website:

> [T]he Pfizer-BioNTech COVID-19 vaccine, utilizes modRNA. modRNA stands for nucleoside-modified messenger RNA and in the synthesis of the RNA used in this vaccine platform, some nucleosides, which are important biological molecules that constitute DNA and RNA, are replaced by modified nucleosides to help ***enhance immune evasion*** and protein production [emphasis ours].[7]

Does modRNA Ever Go Away?

Enhance immune evasion indeed. The effect of a substitution for one of mRNA's nucleotides is profound. Swapping pseudouridine for uridine causes modRNA to resist the expected rapid enzymatic breakdown seen with mRNA. The substitute molecule also shields modRNA from immune system attack, prolonging its life in circulation throughout the body.

This immune evasion is proving to be very successful–perhaps too successful. One study found modRNA and Spike protein hiding out in lymph nodes weeks after injection, not rapidly breaking down as promoted by the CDC and manufacturers.[8]

It is not known if modRNA ever completely clears from the body, continuing to generate toxic Spike proteins that no longer confer protection against SARS-CoV-2 variants.

An August 2023 study found Spike protein in the blood, saliva, urine, and lung fluids of people six months post-COVID-19 vaccine, suggesting mRNA may persist in some cells for extended periods of time or the body has trouble clearing excess Spike proteins, or perhaps both.[9]

As was discussed in Chapter 4, COVID-19, Spike proteins are extremely toxic to the lining of blood vessels and multiple organ systems, including the brain, heart, lungs, and blood. Their continued production due to the elusiveness of modRNA may underlie the large number of well-documented COVID-19 severe adverse events.

modRNA Causes Junk Protein Production

The substitution of pseudouridine for natural uridine in modRNA has another potentially dangerous consequence. As modRNA translates its genetic code to the protein manufacturing systems inside a cell, the presence of pseudouridine occasionally triggers a glitch in reading the code, referred to as "frameshifting."[10]

Frameshifting causes the protein-manufacturing apparatus to misread the genetic code, resulting in production of a junk protein.

Junk protein is just that: a protein that has no function yet may be viewed by the immune system as a foreign invader that needs to be destroyed. The subsequent immune reaction is inflammatory and may exacerbate the known toxicity of modRNA in the vaccinated.

Researchers at Cambridge University recently confirmed that 25% to 30% of patients who received the Pfizer mRNA vaccine experienced an unintended immune response in the form of antibody production against frame-shifted Spike proteins. This means that vaccinated persons are forming antibodies against random proteins caused by the frame-shifting, which can lead to an unwanted inflammatory response, including an autoimmune reaction.[11]

Lipid Nanoparticles (LNPs)

LNPs are essential to deliver modRNA and saRNA to the cells, but are they safe?

On its own, modRNA containing the genetic code for a particular protein has difficulty passing through cell walls. For modRNA to produce the desired protein, it must enter the cell and take control of its protein manufacturing apparatus. A delivery system is essential to carry modRNA to the cell surface and facilitate uptake and release of modRNA inside the cell.

LNPs were selected by researchers to encapsulate modRNA because of their ability to evade immune system attack and efficiency at passing through cell membranes. They are, for all intents and purposes, a molecular Trojan horse. LNPs can even penetrate blood vessel-organ interfaces usually resistant to vaccines or even viruses, such as the blood-brain barrier and the placenta.

Unfortunately, LNPs are toxic and can themselves trigger inflammatory-related adverse events and anaphylaxis.

Back in the 1990s when the mRNA platform technology was being developed, one of the inventors, Robert Malone, MD, abandoned LNPs due to their toxicity.[12] This lesson appears lost on Malone's successors, who continued development of mRNA applications using LNPs.

One such successor was Stéphane Bancel, CEO of Moderna, who stated in 2016:

> Delivery — actually getting RNA into cells — has long bedeviled the whole field. On their own, RNA molecules have a hard time reaching their targets. They work better if they're wrapped up in a delivery mechanism, such as nanoparticles made of lipids. But those nanoparticles can lead to dangerous side effects, especially if a patient has to take repeated doses over months or years.[13]

Despite these concerns, Moderna joined Pfizer as one of the first two manufacturers of COVID-19 mRNA vaccines that used lipid nanoparticle carriers.

Vaccine manufacturers have now conceded that the carrier technology used by their vaccines can be toxic. A paper published in 2024 by Moderna scientists found that the lipid nanoparticles used in its COVID-19 mRNA vaccine can be toxic and might be the root cause of many of the side-effects experienced by people post-vaccination.[14] These include, according to the authors, "heart inflammation and severe allergic shock, . . . most likely triggered by PEGlyated lipid nanoparticles."

As noted below, PEG is polyethylene glycol which can be highly reactogenic (can cause adverse immune reactions).

LNP Toxicity

LNPs are known to be toxic to DNA through the release of reactive oxygen molecules that penetrate the cell nucleus.[15] The particles are coated with polyethylene glycol (PEG), which helps to stabilize the LNPs and keeps them from clumping. However, PEG can trigger anaphylactic allergic reaction, GI distress, electrolyte imbalances, and can be neurotoxic.[16]

LNPs are also known to activate the complement (inflammatory) system and stimulate the secretion of pro-inflammatory cytokines.[17] Complement and cytokines are part of the innate or immediate response component of the immune system. Overstimulation from LNPs can precipitate an overly aggressive immune response that can result in life-threatening side effects.

Several studies describe inflammatory-related adverse events following modRNA injections, including stroke, pericarditis, and myocarditis.[18,19,20]

LNPs Are Widely Distributed

Despite what the public was told about the COVID-19 vaccination staying in the arm and rapidly breaking down, LNPs disperse throughout the body within hours of injection.

Pfizer knew this in advance of FDA's Emergency Use Authorization. "In summary," Pfizer wrote about their own vaccine uptake and distribution study, "over 48 hours, the LNP distributed mainly to **liver, adrenal glands, spleen and ovaries,** with maximum concentrations observed at 8–48 hours post-dose (emphasis ours)."[21]

So much for modRNA vaccine injection localizing to the arm and posing no risk to other organ systems. The observation of LNPs in the reproductive system was a harbinger of the disastrous effects later observed on fertility and pregnancy (see Chapter 19, Pregnancy and Vaccines).

The safety of LNPs as a delivery vehicle remains unproven. Clearly, more research is needed on the safety and toxicity of these compounds before their further use as a vaccine transport vehicle. No child should be subjected to the risk LNPs pose to their developing organ systems.

Why modRNA Vaccines Are So Toxic to Immature Immune Systems

Maternal antibodies

Newborns have maternal antibodies for about the first six to twelve months of life. After that, they become reliant on their own immune capability to respond to infections. Immature immune systems must spend the first few years learning how to adapt to external threats from viruses, bacteria, fungi, and so forth.

Innate (Rapid Response) & Adaptive (Memory) Immune System

Infants have all the tools necessary to develop fully functional immune systems, but it takes exposure to real-world threats to mature. These tools include a rapid response system to active infections known as innate immunity, and a longer-term, memory system known as adaptive immunity.

The *innate system* identifies a foreign invader, mounts an initial defense, and calls for backup from the adaptive immune system through chemical signals. In turn, antibodies are produced specific to the antigens found on the foreign invaders, allowing for their destruction.

The *adaptive system* serves as a library of potential threats, storing the memory of previous invaders in specialized immune cells that can rapidly respond to future infections. The adaptive system is also highly flexible with built-in redundancy, responding to countless variations of previous threats.

The adaptive system can effectively respond to thousands of variants of a particular pathogen by identifying viral components that are less likely to mutate over time.

On the other hand, antibody measurements recorded during testing of the earlier bivalent childhood COVID-19 vaccine trials (since removed from market) refer to bursts of antibody production that peak and then go away after a few weeks or months.

Although antibody measurements were used as a proxy for vaccine effectiveness, antibody responses do not necessarily correlate with disease prevention. Moreover, the observed immune response was non-neutralizing (also called non-sterilizing), meaning it didn't prevent the virus from entering cells and replicating.

modRNA vaccine-induced immunity is directed at a single antigen. In the case of COVID-19 vaccine, this was the Spike or S protein region of the SARS-CoV-2 virus. Mutations to this region in circulating viruses help evade a sterilizing immune response to new variants from the vaccine, making reinfection more likely.

Natural Immunity

In contrast to vaccine-induced immunity, natural immunity will recognize scores of antigens and other molecular markers on the virus and mount a vigorous immune response, making reinfection or serious infection less likely.

Natural immunity from infection by one respiratory virus teaches the young immune system to prepare for other types of respiratory viruses that carry similar chemical signatures, and not just variants of a single virus like SARS-CoV-2.

In this way, a young adaptive immune system library of defense tools is built and becomes robust and cross-reactive to a variety of threats that have yet to be encountered.

Learning to Differentiate Invader from Self

An essential part of the learning process of young immune systems is the ability to differentiate foreign invaders from self.

Viruses often cloak themselves with surface proteins and other compounds that resemble host cells so they can hide from the immune system. Many respiratory viruses share a similar cloaking chemical signature.

A child's immune system must learn not to attack the body's own cells, mistakenly thinking they are infectious agents. Essentially, immature immune systems need to know when to turn off as much as when to turn on.

Immune system confusion about chemical signatures on pathogens versus host cells may trigger auto-immune disorders such as diabetes, rheumatoid arthritis, and multiple sclerosis. This happens when the immune system attacks specific host cell types, resulting in destruction of native cells.

How modRNA Vaccines Like COVID-19 Damage Young Immune Systems

Vaccine-generated antibodies, obtained from either maternal transmission of a vaccinated mom to the fetus or from direct childhood immunization, bind tightly to the SARS-CoV-2 Spike or S-protein (called high affinity). These antibodies outcompete adaptive system antibodies, but as mentioned are non-sterilizing (don't prevent infection and replication).

Consequently, the child's immature immune system is deprived of the "training" it needs to identify and neutralize future variants. If vaccine antibody generation is constrained by response to Spike (S) protein only, for example, the adaptive system may not build a full defensive library to include responses to all the other viral protein sites which are less likely to mutate.

Response to Other Viruses Affected

Viruses often share markers that a developed immune system can identify from previous, unrelated infections, allowing them to mount a more vigorous response. Developing immune systems exposed to limited viral markers because of modRNA vaccination may be less likely to mount a robust immune response to other respiratory viruses. This makes children less capable of fighting off common viruses and more likely to develop chronic viral infections.

Immune Imprinting

As discussed, the adaptive immune system is a critical component of protective immunity. Exposure to a single viral antigen such as the modRNA-generated Spike protein might limit the generation of new immune responses. Essentially, new variants may be capable of evading a neutralizing immune response if protective immunity was trained on a single protein.[22]

The resulting narrowly focused immunity is referred to as immune imprinting (sometimes called original antigenic sin or OAS). OAS may result in several immune system impairments.

Immune imprinting and lack of development of neutralizing antibodies increases the infectiousness of the virus to the vaccinated child as well as vaccinated and boosted adults. Immune imprinting may explain why the greater the number of COVID-19 vaccinations previously received, the higher the risk of contracting COVID-19, according to a study from the Cleveland Clinic.[23]

Conclusion

ModRNA vaccines are a failed technology that have not been proven safe or effective in children. modRNA resists natural breakdown by the immune system and can persist in the body for weeks to months or longer, generating dangerous Spike proteins. LNP carriers are known to be toxic and do not remain at the injection site. They disperse modRNA throughout the body, including to the reproductive organs and brain. The long-term consequences of modRNA on fertility, neurodevelopment, and the immune system are unknown.

Until there are definitive, multi-year clinical trials that demonstrate both safety and effectiveness of modRNA vaccines compared with a true placebo, parents and caregivers are cautioned about subjecting children to this unproven technology.

CHAPTER 18

Gardasil® and HPV—High Risk, Low Reward

On June 8, 2006, the FDA licensed the first HPV-vaccine, Gardasil® (Merck), to be used primarily for girls and women between the ages of 9 and 26.[1] Subsequently, the CDC recommended routine HPV vaccination at ages eleven to twelve as the primary measure to protect children from "certain cancers later in life."[2] They also advise that, if children start their vaccine series on or after 15 years of age, three doses should be given over six months. Further, the CDC recommends that females through the age of 26 and males through age 21 should have "catch-up vaccinations."[3]

Background

Human papillomavirus (HPV) is a common sexually transmitted disease (STD) that is known to be highly contagious.[4] Some types of HPV may increase the risk for developing certain types of cancer, especially cervical.[5] The CDC heavily promotes these vaccinations stating that they protect people from getting infected with specific cancer-causing HPV type strains.

HPV is characterized by warts or lesions that may develop into cancer. Currently, there are over 600 strains of HPV, with twelve identified as "high-risk HPV" types.[6] Of these twelve, two are found in most HPV-related cancers: HPV 16 and HPV 18.[7]

HPV and Cervical Cancer

The National Cancer Institute (NCI) states that "virtually all cervical cancer" is caused by the HPV virus.[8] NCI also affirms that, in most people, the immune system clears the infection (typically within a year or two) without causing cancer.[9]

The average age of HPV-related cancer diagnosis is between 50 and 68 years.[10] Cervical cancer is the most common type of HPV-associated cancer, and it is usually diagnosed earlier than the others, at age 50. Globally, the median age of cervical cancer diagnosis is 53, with the average age at death being 59.[11]

Type of Cancer	Average age of diagnosis
Cervical	50
Vaginal	68
Vulvar	67
Anal	63 (women), 61 (men)
Mouth/Throat	63 (women), 61 (men)

Average age (years) that HPV-associated cancer occurs in women and men, according to the CDC.[12]

CDC's HPV-Vaccine Campaign

HPV vaccine promotional campaigns target millions of preadolescent and adolescent children for whom the risk of developing cervical cancer is remote. School-age children at no risk of developing HPV-related cancers are being vaccinated with multiple doses during their primary years of sexual development. Some cancers, such as vaginal and vulvar, are typically diagnosed around age sixty-eight, a fifty-five-year gap between vaccination and the potential onset of cancer.

According to the National Cancer Institute, the rate of new cervical cancer cases is 7.7 per 100,000 women per year.[13] This means that in any given year, .008% of all women in the United States are diagnosed with cervical cancer. The low incidence stands in stark contrast to promotional messaging that vaccines are essential to curb an epidemic of HPV-related cancers.

The central message of the promotional campaigns is to protect yourself and protect others you care about from a cancer-causing infection. This is a compelling and emotional appeal, but it is a distortion of reality. The human immune system and regular Pap smears with proper follow-up of abnormal results are generally all the protection needed to prevent cervical cancer except for those who suffer from a rare genetic predisposition or are immune suppressed.

Considering the unlikelihood of adolescents and teens developing cervical and other HPV-related cancers, one would think that HPV vaccine risks should be near zero. Unfortunately, this is not the case.

Vaccine Effectiveness

HPV vaccines have *never* been shown to prevent cancer. Based on a Relative Risk Reduction calculation, HPV vaccines are 98% to 100% effective at preventing *precancerous changes* to the most superficial layer of cervical cells, the epithelia, over a three-year period.[14] It should be duly noted that precancerous changes are not the same as cancer.

However, using clinical study data provided in the Gardasil®9 package insert, the Absolute Risk Reduction is roughly 1.5%.[15] In other words, a woman of average risk reduces her chances of precancerous changes by just 1.5% from vaccination. Even accepting the 98% to 100% risk reduction numbers, it is not possible to correlate inhibition of precancerous changes in the cervical epithelium with cancer prevention due to two main factors.

First, the average lag time between precancerous cells and the diagnosis of cancer is over twenty years.[16] It is not possible to assess vaccine efficacy with respect to cancer prevention within a three-year time frame.

Second, around 98–99% of precancerous conditions will resolve on their own.[17,18] Most are the result of inflammation or infection. Around three million women have abnormal Pap tests each year, yet fewer than 1% will be diagnosed with cancer.[19] Moreover, cervical cancer is generally regarded as treatable and curable, particularly if diagnosed at an early stage.

Researchers Express Caution

In an editorial that accompanied the key HPV vaccine study cited above, editors wisely raised another issue perhaps more important than the clinical results. They stated,

> We must also carefully monitor for unintended adverse consequences of vaccination. For example, when selective immunologic pressure is applied with vaccination, the potential exists for non vaccine-related strains [of HPV] to emerge as important oncogenic serotypes.[20]

Their concerns were justified. HPV strains not covered by the vaccines are posing new cancer threats, as discussed below.

HPV-Vaccine Safety Examined

In the two and a half years immediately following Gardasil® approval in 2006, over 12,000 adverse events were reported to the FDA's Vaccine Adverse Event Reporting System (VAERS). Among these reports were 772 serious adverse events, including Guillain-Barré syndrome, motor neuron disease, and pancreatitis; there were also 32 deaths with an average age of 18.[21]

Since 2006, 136 million doses of HPV vaccine (and counting) have been given to children and young adults in the United States. In this period, three vaccines have been developed and licensed by the FDA:

- Gardasil® (stopped marketing in 2017)
- Cervarix (approved in 2009 and withdrawn from the market in 2016)
- Gardasil®9 (approved in 2014)

Gardasil®9, the only HPV vaccine currently approved for use in the US, protects against nine HPV types (strains), including 6, 11, 16, 18, 31, 33, 45, 52, and 58.[22]

The CDC assures the public that HPV vaccines "are very safe" with the benefits outweighing the potential risks of the vaccine.[23] They also report that each of the three vaccines that have been used in children and adults were extensively safety tested in clinical trials. The CDC asserts that in these trials, each "HPV vaccine was found to be safe and effective."[24]

Despite these assurances, HPV vaccination side effects are common and include headaches, nausea, dizziness, and fainting.[25,26] Further, HPV vaccine has been shown to increase the risk for developing chronic immune, neurological, and pain disorders, among other serious adverse events.[27] Plausible associations exist between HPV vaccines and autoimmune disorders, premature ovarian failure, Guillain-Barré Syndrome, and postural orthostatic tachycardia syndrome (POTS).[28,29]

Further evidence linking autoimmune disorders with HPV vaccine was published in the journal Vaccine in early 2024. Researchers found that girls and young women between nine and nineteen years of age had a markedly elevated risk of developing one of four autoimmune disorders within one year. These included rheumatoid arthritis, juvenile idiopathic arthritis, thrombocytopenic purpura (low platelets leading to bruising and internal bleeding), and thyrotoxicosis (excessive thyroid hormone causing rapid pulse, weakness, anxiety, etc.).[30]

Gardasil®9 has not been evaluated for the potential to cause carcinogenicity or genotoxicity (damage to genes), nor has it been studied for its impact on fertility.[31]

Aluminum and HPV Vaccine Clinical Trials

During the original Gardasil® clinical trials, Merck failed to disclose that the placebo comparison group contained an aluminum adjuvant (an agent that enhances the effect of the vaccine) known as amorphous aluminum hydroxyphosphate sulfate (AAHS), and not saline.[32] AAHS is Merck's proprietary adjuvant formulation and has never been safety tested in humans.

The absence of a true placebo makes detection of a safety concern difficult. The presence of AAHS in the placebo arm of the study gives the impression that the vaccine is as safe as the placebo, whereas both groups suffered many serious medical adverse events.[33]

Aluminum in the form of AAHS is also an active ingredient in Gardasil®9.[34] The amount of AAHS in Gardasil® 9 is more than double that of the original Gardasil® vaccine.

Studies in humans and animals have shown that the types of aluminum used in vaccines are toxic and can cause nerve damage, neurological disorders, autoimmune disorders, and death.[35,36] In contrast to ingested aluminum, injected aluminum compounds are readily absorbed and can cross the blood-brain barrier, the protective shield that protects the brain from harmful toxins. The metal has been shown in studies to impair motor and cognitive function while increasing risk for developing a neurodegenerative disorder (i.e., Alzheimer's disease).[37] See Chapter 2, First, Do No Harm for more information about aluminum toxicity.

Connecting Symptoms With Biological Markers

A 2022 Danish HPV vaccine study examined the links between HPV vaccination and autoimmunity over the course of several years. The result? Girls and young women experiencing long-term, vaccine-related complications exhibited the same biological markers found in autoimmune disorders.[38]

The top four symptoms reported by 90% of study participants were fatigue, dizziness, cognitive dysfunction, and headache, which are typical autoimmune reactions. More than 80% described their fatigue as moderate or severe. Over two thirds described trouble sleeping, nausea, abdominal pain, heart palpitations, and muscle weakness.[39]

In addition to their symptoms, the study group exhibited biological markers of an inflammatory response. One test used as a key biomarker in rheumatic diseases was significantly higher than in the control group (59% versus 25%). In another test that measures certain kinds of autoantibodies (antibodies mistakenly directed against the body's own structures), 92% of the symptomatic group had autoantibodies versus 19% of controls.[40]

Gates Foundation, Government, and Funding the HPV-Vaccine

Since the HPV vaccine was first approved, the United States Government has heavily promoted its use. The government spent $300 million in a massive vaccination program, including the award of more than fifty grants totaling over $40 million to universities, health-care systems, and departments of public health to increase HPV vaccine uptake.[41,42]

Promoting the vaccine is not just centered in the United States. The Gates Foundation gave $600 million to fund Gavi, The Vaccine Alliance with a goal of vaccinating 86 million girls in low-income countries.[43] Gavi partners not only with the Bill and Melinda Gates Foundation, but also vaccine manufacturers, World Bank, WHO, and private sector partners.[44] The European Medicines Agency (EMA) has produced publications in an organized effort to dismiss negative publicity.[45,46]

Expansion of HPV Target Market

US Health and Human Services, non-governmental organizations (NGOs), and vaccine manufacturers have recently begun promoting the vaccine to people twenty-seven years of age and older in order to expand the market of eligibles. The push may reflect concerns about the relatively low rate of HPV vaccine uptake among adolescents and early teens.[47]

In 2019, the Advisory Committee on Immunization Practices (ACIP) officially recommended that physicians discuss HPV vaccination with their patients aged 27 to 45 years.[48] This recommendation was made despite evidence of negative vaccine efficacy if someone was already infected.

Negative Vaccine Efficacy

Merck's own Gardasil® clinical trials found that vaccinating an already infected person with a vaccine-covered strain increases the risk of precancerous changes to the cervix by between 33% and 44.6%.[49]

More than 25% of women ages 30–39 years will test positive for HPV,[50] posing a potential health risk for older vaccinees should they be infected with one of the nine strains covered by the vaccine. As such, follow-up studies are essential to assure the safety of HPV vaccination in those over 27 who may have active HPV infection.

HPV-Vaccine Adverse Events Underreported

A 2009 study published in *JAMA Network* details adverse event reports following vaccination with the first-released Gardasil®.[51] According to the study, there were a total of 12,454 adverse events reported to VAERS following HPV vaccination over a two-year period (2006-2008).[52]

The majority of these reports were submitted by Merck (68%), and 772 involved a seriously adverse event, including anaphylaxis, deep vein thrombosis (blood clot), Guillain-Barré syndrome (ascending paralysis), convulsions, pulmonary embolism, pancreatitis, and autoimmune disorders. Thirty-two deaths were also reported, with twenty verified through clinical autopsies.[53]

A subsequent study published in *Science, Public Health Policy, and the Law* examined the data from the Merck reports and determined that the adverse event percentage of 6.2%, was exceedingly low.[54] The study authors asked a panel of volunteer, licensed physicians to rate the VAERS reports. The physicians rated 24.2% of the adverse events as "serious" using legal criteria as defined by the statutory Code of Federal Regulation, or CFR.[55] These criteria include:[56]

- Death
- Life-threatening adverse event
- Inpatient hospitalization or prolongation of existing hospitalization
- Persistent or significant incapacity or substantial disruption of the ability to conduct normal life functions
- Congenital anomaly/birth defect

Cervical (Pap) Screening, Not Vaccination, Lowers Incidence and Risk

Regarding the promotional theme of protecting oneself and others, HPV vaccination has had virtually no impact on the rate of cervical cancer in the 19 years since the vaccine was first approved. In 2005, the year before Gardasil® came on to the market, the rate of new cervical cancer cases was 7.9 per 100,000 women per year, compared with the current rate of 7.7 per 100,000 women per year.[57] In the 19 years since Gardasil® was released the needle has barely moved.

The National Cancer Institute's SEER program compared how many women died of cervical cancer before Gardasil® was first introduced to the present. They found that the cancer had been declining at a steady rate for several years before the vaccine was released, primarily because of increased Pap screening.[58]

This 2022 study asked the question, "Does vaccination protect against human papillomavirus-related cancers?" using data drawn from the United States National Health and Nutrition Examination Survey (2011–2018).[59] In this cross-sectional study, the researchers did *not* find a protective relationship between HPV-vaccination with HPV-related cancers.[60]

According to Johns Hopkins School of Public Health, cervical cancer is rare because the majority of cancers are detected by screening when they are still pre-cancers, and the decrease in the number of cancer cases is due to "successes in cancer screening."[61]

Government Task Force Agrees

The US Preventive Services Task Force (USPSTF) states that widespread cervical cancer screening in women aged 21-65 "substantially reduces cervical cancer incidence and mortality."[62] The USPSTF also affirms that the screening campaign is the primary reason why the number of deaths from cervical cancer has declined from 2.8 to 2.3 per 100,000 women.[63]

Risk Factors for HPV Infection

Sex before the age of sixteen and having sex with multiple partners pose a greater risk for HPV infection and developing cervical cancer. Other risk factors are HIV infection and smoking. A 2020 study published in Oncology Letters reported that having multiple partners and engaging in unprotected sex can change the healthy ecology of a woman's vagina and increase her risk for HPV infection and associated cervical cancer.[64] Refraining from unprotected sex with multiple partners is the best protection against HPV-related cancer.

Backfilling With High-Risk HPV Strains

Viruses survive by mutating to overcome barriers to their survival, including vaccines. Vaccine manufacturers respond with new versions of their vaccines.[65] In the case of HPV vaccines, Gardasil® expanded its covered strains from four to nine. However, it is often the vaccines themselves that create the conditions for evolution of new strains.[66]

Peer-reviewed studies have shown that HPV strains that are suppressed by the vaccine may lead to opening of an ecological niche that is backfilled by more virulent strains, a phenomenon known as type replacement.[67,68,69] Some previously classified lower-risk strains not covered by the vaccines have been reclassified as high-risk HPV types as they backfill for suppressed strains.[70]

Conclusion

HPV vaccines have not been shown to prevent cancer or to reduce the amount of cervical or other HPV-related cancers in vaccine-eligible populations. The human immune system and regular Pap smears remain the most effective methods for preventing cervical cancer. Modifiable risk factors include engaging in sexual intercourse before age sixteen, multiple sexual partners, and smoking.

The risks of HPV vaccine are considerable, including various neurological, cardiac, reproductive and immunological disorders. Studies have shown that HPV strains that are suppressed by the vaccine may lead to backfilling by equally virulent strains.

Another potential risk is that women may decide to skip regular Pap screening, assuming vaccination protects them from HPV infection. This is a particular concern for women who do not regularly visit a provider.[71]

The government's aggressive promotion of vaccines and the large expansion by age of target groups is reminiscent of COVID-19 promotions. Questions about vaccine effectiveness and safety should give pause to government agencies, who should insist on longer duration clinical trials and use of true placebo groups for comparison of serious adverse events.

What is not in doubt is the effectiveness of regular Pap screening and leading a healthy lifestyle, including limiting the number of unprotected sexual encounters.

The CDC's recommendation for cervical cancer screening can be found here:

CHAPTER 19

Vaccines and Pregnancy: Risky Business

Neither Safe nor Effective

The CDC recommends women receive several vaccines during pregnancy to protect not only themselves, but their unborn child. These include Flu, TdaP, RSV, and COVID-19 vaccines–all of which the CDC claims to be safe for a pregnant woman and her baby.

Vaccine	1st Trimester	2nd Trimester	3rd Trimester
Tdap	X	X	✓
Flu (inactivated)	✓	✓	✓
COVID-19	✓	✓	✓
RSV	X	X	✓

Recommended vaccines (✓) per trimester as advised by the CDC.

With the premise that a baby gets disease protection from their mother during pregnancy, the CDC states that getting these vaccines allows the mother to pass antibodies on to their unborn child. The CDC also assures that these four vaccines are safe for pregnant women and their babies.

All mothers and parents-to-be deserve access to more information than CDC assurances so they can make informed decisions about vaccinations during pregnancy.

Influenza Vaccine

In 2019, ICAN (Informed Consent Action Network) asked for a copy of each report from the FDA of clinical trials that were used to support the safety of vaccines during pregnancy. The federal regulating agency was required by law to supply this information under the FOIA (Freedom of Information Act).

When the FDA failed to respond to the request, a lawsuit followed that suggested they had never licensed a vaccine to be used for pregnant women. The FDA responded to this inquiry stating, "We have no records responsive to your requests." This means the FDA had *no records* of any clinical trial that a vaccine was ever tested on pregnant women to ensure its safety.[1]

Are Flu Vaccines Safe for Pregnant Women?

A 2021 *JAMA* study claimed that vaccines posed no risk for pregnant women.[2] The study authors posed the question: "Is seasonal influenza vaccination in pregnancy associated with adverse childhood outcomes?" Their answer was that there was no *significant* association with adverse childhood outcomes among vaccinated offspring. However, according to Brian Hooker, PhD, the researchers got it wrong.

In the study, out of a cohort of 28,255 children born in Nova Scotia, 36% were exposed to the influenza vaccine during gestation. The researchers followed the children's health for an average of 3.6 years and concluded there were no associated adverse outcomes reported (including asthma, upper and lower respiratory infections, gastrointestinal infections, abnormal tissue growths, and hearing or vision loss).

The study failed to consider several factors when drawing this conclusion. The researchers relied only on ER and hospital data and ignored outpatient records that recorded higher rates of GI and lower respiratory infection. Authors also claimed no difference in outcomes between the vaccinated and unvaccinated, despite ear infections occurring at a higher rate in the vaccinated group. Lastly, the all-cause injuries (meaning injuries from any cause) in the control diagnosis group showed significantly higher numbers in the maternally vaccinated children as compared to the unvaccinated.

Study: Spontaneous Abortions

In 2017, the CDC published a seismic study that directly linked spontaneous abortions in women to flu vaccines.[3] In a review of data from the 2010-11 and 2011-12 flu seasons, women who were vaccinated with the inactivated influenza virus had twice the chance of a spontaneous abortion within twenty-eight days of receiving the inoculation. The most alarming statistic to come out of this study was that in women who received the H1N1 vaccine, there was a 7.7 times greater incidence of a miscarriage in the twenty-eight days following the shot. Despite the threat to the unborn child, the CDC still recommended all flu vaccines that contain the H1N1 strain for use during pregnancy.

Other Related Risks: Inflammation, Autism, and Diabetes

Inflammation

Beyond the risk of a spontaneous abortion, there are several other increased risks from taking the flu vaccine. A primary impetus in giving the vaccine is to promote an immune response, which, starting with the innate (quick response) immune system, by definition is inflammatory.

Inflammation is a natural part of the body's defense system, helping the body to recognize harmful foreign substances (such as a virus) and begin healing and recovery.[4]

In utero, inflammation can also have serious consequences, including an increased risk for psychiatric disorders and autism. The trivalent influenza virus vaccination has been shown in studies to cause a measurable inflammatory response which is associated with adverse health outcomes for the mother and child.[5]

Autism

One of these adverse health outcomes is autism. A 2014 study reinforces the notion that inflammation during pregnancy, regardless of whether from vaccines, is associated with autism.[6] Alan Brown, M.D. and his colleagues found that of the 1.2 million pregnant women studied, elevated CRP levels were associated with a 43% greater risk of having a child with autism. Keep in mind that CRP, or C-reactive protein, is the same marker of inflammation that increases after flu vaccination.

A 2021 study also concluded that maternal immune activation plays a significant role in the pathogenesis of autism. Inflammation and associated cellular stress have been reported in the brain tissues of individuals diagnosed with autism spectrum disorder. The study authors stated the inflammatory processes (like those that happen after flu vaccination) cause a "self-perpetuating vicious cycle that leads to abnormalities in brain development and behavior."[7]

Gestational Diabetes and Eclampsia

Gestational diabetes, preeclampsia, and eclampsia are serious conditions that can develop during pregnancy, posing a risk for both mother and baby. Preeclampsia is characterized by high blood pressure, edema or water retention, and protein in the urine. This condition can cause a number of problems for a pregnant woman and baby, including low birth weight and risk of hemorrhage during childbirth. It can also lead to eclampsia (dangerous seizures that are life-threatening). Gestational diabetes is a form of diabetes that only develops in pregnancy and is associated with elevated blood sugar levels that can lead to an increased risk for C-section, preeclampsia, and depression.

Another study published in the British Medical Journal reported that the influenza vaccine increased the risk for gestational diabetes and life-threatening eclampsia.[8] In 2014, Giuseppe Traversa and colleagues assessed maternal, fetal, and neonatal outcomes of women given the influenza A/H1N1 vaccine. The outcomes of over 86,000 pregnancies revealed that vaccinated women had significantly higher rates of gestational diabetes and eclampsia.

Birth Defects

In a 2016 study, Chambers et al. found a moderately elevated risk for birth defects among children born to mothers who received one flu vaccine during the 2010-2014 flu seasons. A closer look at the study revealed that exposure to the vaccine during the first trimester was associated with nearly twice as many major birth defects than among the unexposed babies (5.7% vs 3.0%).

Marginally Effective Outcomes

Each year, influenza vaccines are formulated based on strains identified months in advance based on global flu surveillance. All flu vaccines in the US are "quadrivalent," meaning they are based on four different flu viruses (two influenza A viruses and two influenza B viruses). The CDC *guesses* which strains will predominate in the US in the coming flu season based on what strains are in circulation in the southern hemisphere six months in advance.

Every year, flu vaccine effectiveness (VE) rarely rises above 50%. For example, the 2021-2022 flu season saw a 16% VE rate and for the 2022-2023 flu season CDC reports a 23% VE rate against hospitalizations for adults aged 18-64 years.[9, 10] When adverse effects from flu vaccines are considered, the risk-to-benefit ratio does not support vaccination for most people. Yet, the push is on each year to get everyone vaccinated.

Do Repeat Vaccinations Increase the Risk?

At least two studies suggest repeated influenza vaccinations increase the risk of influenza infection. The latest was co-authored by the CDC's own investigators who found that there was an 11% increase in the rate of infection following vaccination for certain strains.[11] The authors speculated about factors that may have contributed to increased risk of infection following repeat vaccination but concluded they "cannot fully explain the increased infection risk in repeat vaccinees compared with non-repeat vaccinees."[12]

This investigation follows a similar report from 2015 when Canadian researchers found those vaccinated during the prior flu season had a 15% increased risk of infection compared to the unvaccinated.[13]

Observation of negative effectiveness has driven some Canadian public health officials to reconsider universal flu vaccine programs. Ontario's former chief medical officer, once a proponent of universal programs stated,

> We should . . . do a very careful rethink of where we are. There's enough new evidence that we should all be troubled enough by . . . our policies. There are more and more unanswered questions about how effective a universal program really is.[14]

Perhaps the experts in the CDC U.S. Flu Vaccine Effectiveness Network should consider these sentiments and acknowledge that, much like with the COVID-19 mRNA vaccines, repeat immunization against the same virus has been shown to diminish an effective antibody immune response.[15]

Profitable Vaccine with Recurring Revenue

While not very effective for most people, influenza vaccines generate steady cash flow year in and year out. Flu vaccines are a big profit center, generating nearly $7 billion in annual revenue and expected to grow to $10 billion by 2028.[16] There has never been a successful vaccine developed to prevent any of the common respiratory viruses that afflict humans–despite billions of research dollars. They simply mutate too quickly. Yet, they remain widely embraced by the public and the medical community. Look for increased promotion of combination influenza-COVID-19 vaccines in an effort to reverse declining sales of the unpopular COVID-19 vaccines.

Conclusion: Influenza Vaccine

On balance, a risk-benefit assessment strongly mitigates against giving the flu vaccine to pregnant women *who are in good health.* The influenza vaccine was never tested on pregnant women prior to approval. The testing since approval in support of its use is equivocal to contradictory. Several studies point strongly to the potential for harm to babies, including an increased risk for autism, gestational diabetes, eclampsia, asthma, and gastrointestinal disorders. Lastly, the flu vaccine is marginally effective (as low as 13%).[17] It is unclear whether influenza vaccination in high-risk pregnancies or for mothers with chronic illnesses offers a better risk-benefit profile.

COVID-19 Vaccine

The CDC states that the COVID vaccines are "unlikely to pose risk for pregnant people."[18] However, the CDC also admits that there is limited information available about the safety of the COVID-19 vaccine. A closer look reveals that the COVID-19 vaccination is risky for not only pregnant people, but for those trying to conceive.

Further, the CDC pushes a vaccine that fails to protect babies and mothers from COVID in the first place. Let's explore how government agencies and professional health and medical organizations push an ineffective vaccine that carries unnecessary risks for mother, baby, and parents-to-be.

ACOG's Vaccine Advocacy

The American College of Obstetricians and Gynecologists (ACOG) claims to be the "premier professional membership organization for obstetricians and gynecologists," counting over sixty thousand members across North and South America. Most obstetricians belong to ACOG and are influenced by its policies.

Confidential documents obtained under a Freedom of Information Act (FOIA) request reveal the potential for undue influence between the federal Health and Human Services (HHS), the Center for Disease Control (CDC), and the American College of Obstetricians and Gynecologists (ACOG).[19]

On April 1, 2021, the Department of Health and Human Services formally introduced the COVID-19 Community Corps, a membership organization formed to promote vaccines to as many people as possible.[20] HHS had a war chest of over $16 billion in grant money to be awarded to non-government organizations (NGOs) to recruit what HHS refers to as "trusted community leaders."

In this campaign, HHS targeted 275 influential NGOs and health and medical organizations, including the AMA, American Academy of Pediatrics, and the ACOG. These organizations, influencers, and individuals could serve as "trusted messengers" to promote the COVID-19 vaccine.

HHS hoped that their vaccine promotion would penetrate even the most sacrosanct of relationships, that between a patient and her doctor. ACOG joined the Community Corps as a founding member, ultimately receiving millions in HHS/CDC grant money. As of 2022, ACOG received grants totaling over $11 million to promote COVID-19 injections.

Maternal COVID Vaccination Fails to Protect Babies

The CDC, HHS, and the ACOG promote COVID-19 vaccines for pregnant women, promising protection for their unborn babies. In fact, the CDC directly states on their "Pregnant and Protected" website that "[w]omen who are vaccinated before or during pregnancy or while breastfeeding are protected from getting very sick; [they also] help protect their babies from serious illness caused by COVID-19."[21]

However, studies show that this statement lacks broad scientific support.

A close look at a study published in *JAMA Network Open* reveals that vaccination during pregnancy has unacceptably low vaccine effectiveness.[22] The study authors looked at a cohort of 7,292 infants aged six months or older to see if they were protected from COVID after vaccination. The results revealed that vaccination before or during pregnancy did not influence babies testing positive with Omicron variant.

Further, Goh and colleagues from the *JAMA* study reported low estimated vaccine effectiveness of 15.4-26.2%, far below the typical threshold for vaccine approval of 50%. Based on this data, vaccine risks appear to outweigh potential benefits.

Pfizer and FDA Hid Data

It was revealed in April 2023 that Pfizer and the FDA knew in early 2021 that the modRNA vaccine caused severe fetal harm and posed risks to breastfed infants.

The information was contained in documents released under court order which would have been otherwise withheld from public view for seventy-five years.[23]

Among the documents released was one titled "Pregnancy and Lactation Cumulative Review" that summarized clinical trial data through February 2021. The information was brought to light by a team of clinicians, attorneys, statisticians, and other volunteers organized by the Daily Clout who combed through thousands of pages of released documents.[24] A copy of the original Pfizer report can be found at this reference.[25]

Clinical trials typically exclude pregnant and lactating women from participating due to the increased risk to developing fetus and child, a practice observed during the Pfizer studies.[26] However, many of the exposures occurred as a result of vaccination prior to or during the first trimester–before women knew they were pregnant or were to become pregnant.

What is revealed in their document is chilling.

Of the 673 cases identified by Pfizer, 458 involved exposure during pregnancy; 54% of these reported adverse events. These include 51 cases of spontaneous abortion, six premature labor and delivery cases (including two newborn deaths), one case of newborn severe respiratory distress, and a case of fetal tachycardia with an irregular heart rate over 180 beats per minute that required early delivery and hospitalization.

Of the 673 cases, 215 involved exposure of infants during breastfeeding. Forty-one of the 215 babies exposed through mother's breast milk suffered a range of adverse events, including fever, rash, irritability, diarrhea, lethargy, vomiting, agitation, and facial paralysis.

Just three days after Pfizer signed off on their internal report, the CDC announced in a White House press briefing that they recommended pregnant people receive a COVID-19 vaccination.[27]

More Evidence for Increased Risk of Spontaneous Abortion

A *New England Journal of Medicine* study titled "Preliminary Findings of mRNA Covid-19 Vaccine Safety in Pregnant Persons" claims to demonstrate the safety of mRNA COVID-19 vaccine during pregnancy. However, researchers used a study design that artificially lowered the rate of spontaneous abortion and stillbirth, augmenting the limited data available on the safety of the vaccine.[28]

The study reported a rate of spontaneous abortion following vaccination no different than that found in the general population. However, a closer look at the data shows that over 80% of trial participants were women vaccinated in their third trimester—well after the highest risk for spontaneous abortion.[29] Had these women been excluded from the study, the rate of spontaneous abortion miscarriage rises significantly above the norm, resulting in a markedly different conclusion about vaccine safety.

Concerns raised by the *NEJM* study about the increased risk of miscarriage following COVID-19 vaccination are supported by findings from a 2023 study published in the *British Journal of Obstetrics and Gynaecology* (*BJOG*).[30] This article *also* purports to show that there was no increase in miscarriage following vaccination.

However, a look at the raw data from the *BJOG* study tells a very different story. Instead of no effect, the raw data reveal a near doubling of the rate of miscarriage in the vaccine group compared with the unvaccinated group. In order to arrive at the original conclusion, the study authors introduced an entirely new and irrelevant detail: the incidence of induced abortions.

It is worth noting that the second author on the study has since left her academic institution, which is heavily government financed, to join Pfizer, another example of the vaccine revolving door.

Vaccine mRNA Spreads to Placenta and Umbilical Cord Blood

A 2024 study published in the *American Journal of Obstetrics and Gynecology* aimed to assess whether COVID-19 vaccine mRNA was present in the placenta and cord blood following maternal vaccination during pregnancy.[31] Pfizer and Moderna animal studies detected the presence of lipid nanoparticles containing COVID-19 mRNA in placental tissues and other fetal organs.[32]

Researchers at NYU School of Medicine wished to determine if such exposure takes place in humans. Vaccine mRNA was detected in two placentas tested as well as in the cord blood of one of the patients (cord blood was not tested in the second patient).

The study authors conclude:

> Our findings suggest that the vaccine mRNA is not localized to the injection site and can spread systemically to the placenta and umbilical cord blood. The detection of the spike protein in the placental tissue indicates the bioactivity of the vaccine mRNA reaching the placenta.
>
> To our knowledge, these two cases demonstrate, for the first time, the ability of the COVID-19 vaccine mRNA to penetrate the fetal-placental barrier and reach the intrauterine environment.[33]

Preconception and Beyond

A 2023 study of preconception concluded that COVID-19 vaccination in either partner at any time before conception is not associated with an increased rate of miscarriage. To arrive at that conclusion, researchers asked couples trying to get pregnant if they had been vaccinated and how many times. Couples were then followed through subsequent pregnancies, comparing the rate of miscarriage between vaccinated and unvaccinated couples.

Everything seemed straightforward until researchers "adjusted" the data to form groups of similar risk for miscarriage. An independent analysis of the data reveals that the researchers excluded those most at risk of miscarriage from the vaccinated group from their analysis.[34] Without explanation, researchers "excluded 75 vaccinated women, most likely to miscarry, for each similarly situated unvaccinated woman."[35]

Another 2023 study published in *Journal of Medical Virology* revealed that newborn babies are 1.78 times more likely to contract Covid-19 during the first six months of life after maternal vaccination compared with unvaccinated mothers.[36] The study was a meta-analysis of 30 previous studies representing over 800,000 pregnancies and undermines the argument that the vaccine protects neonates.

Elevated Risk of Myocardial Injuries in Women

A 2023 study titled "Sex-specific differences in myocardial injury incidence after COVID-19 mRNA-1273 booster vaccination" followed 777 health-care workers who had been vaccinated with a Moderna booster.[37] The authors reported a high incidence of myocardial injury markers three days after vaccination, especially in women. Twenty of 22 participants who experienced myocardial injuries were female. The study concluded that myocardial injury was more common than previously thought and occurred more frequently in women than men.

Pregnancy is accompanied by remarkable changes in the cardiovascular system.[38] These include increases in heart rate, cardiac output (the volume of blood pumped from the heart), fluid volume, and changes in blood pressure. For example, by the fifth week of pregnancy, the cardiac output increases to 50% above pre-pregnancy levels.[39]

All these factors combined place quite a stress on the woman's body which can uncover underlying cardiovascular disease.[40] In fact, the leading cause of maternal deaths (33%) is cardiovascular disease, with over 50% of these deaths occurring postpartum.[41]

Considering the female predominance of myocardial injury as noted in this study, pregnant women may be at elevated risk of injury and death from mRNA COVID-19 vaccine.

Conclusion: COVID-19

Federal agencies like the HHS and CDC along with professional organizations such as the ACOG remain in full support of vaccination prior to and during all trimesters of pregnancy. The evidence from multiple studies is equivocal at best, and some study designs resulted in misleading results, creating a false sense of COVID-19 safety during pregnancy and subsequent neonatal immunity. Based on the available information, the safety and efficacy of COVID-19 vaccination during pregnancy remain uncertain.

Tdap Vaccine

In 2012, the CDC began recommending the Tdap vaccine (tetanus toxoid, reduced diphtheria toxoid and acellular pertussis) for pregnant women during their third trimester. They currently recommend that the vaccine should be given during each pregnancy, stating that women can give their babies protection against pertussis (whooping cough) before they are born.[42,43]

The FDA's original approval of the two Tdap brands (Boostrix® and Adacel®) in the mid-2000s was as a booster for teens and adults, and the product inserts state that Tdap should be given during pregnancy only "when benefit outweighs risk." At the time of the 2011 recommendation, no prelicensure studies of Tdap safety during pregnancy were available, so most of the (largely unpublished) data used to justify the recommendation came from post-licensure pregnancy surveillance studies conducted by vaccine manufacturers.

CDC Advocates for Tdap Vaccination During Third Trimester

According to the CDC, infants are most vulnerable to pertussis infection during their first six months as they build immunity from vaccination. Consequently, the CDC recommends mothers receive third trimester vaccination to protect the child during the first six months of life by the passive transfer of maternal antibodies. CDC claims vaccination during pregnancy prevents 78% of cases and 90% of hospitalizations in infants younger than two months.

The CDC's Tdap recommendation is consistent with the other three vaccines also promoted during pregnancy: RSV, influenza, and COVID-19. Common to all these recommendations is the absence of published, peer-reviewed, controlled clinical trials regarding vaccine safety and effectiveness during pregnancy.

Additionally, the CDC's claim of third-trimester vaccine Tdap effectiveness was not the result of a prospective clinical trial in pregnancy. Rather, the CDC's recommendation was based on reanalysis of four previous observational studies which used a non-US formulation.

Put plainly, the CDC extracted data from old retrospective, observational studies, then recombined the data and subjected it to various statistical analyses to arrive at their estimate of vaccine effectiveness using a vaccine not available in the US.

Weak Evidence for Safety and Effectiveness During Pregnancy

For one of two Tdap brands (Boostrix®), a single clinical trial of a few hundred pregnant women (341 in Tdap group, 346 placebo) was used to justify the safety of the vaccine during pregnancy.[44] The trial included no long-term safety data and was never published in a peer-reviewed journal.

Adacel®, a second brand of Tdap, cites a single reanalysis of retrospective data obtained from an unrelated study as the basis for estimating vaccine effectiveness.[45] The reanalysis was conducted on a total of 271 cases of which 32 were given Adacel during the third trimester. Again, there was no prospective, controlled, randomized trial cited as evidence of safety or effectiveness.

Suppression of Infant Immune Response to Pertussis

A study of immune responses of infants born to mothers who received Tdap during pregnancy found diminished antibody responses to pertussis antigens compared with infants whose mothers received placebo during pregnancy.[46] The clinical implications of this finding are unknown but certainly run contrary to the prevailing concept of a protective shield while an infant builds immunity.

Increases Risk for Congenital Birth Defects

Tdap vaccine is recommended in the third trimester only in pregnant women, presumably to protect the fetus during the first two trimesters from vaccine toxicity. This is a justifiable concern. A 2023 study published in peer-reviewed *Infectious Diseases and Therapy* reveals the potential for an elevated risk of congenital birth defects attributed to the vaccine.[47]

The study titled "Investigating Tetanus, Diphtheria, Acellular Pertussis Vaccination During Pregnancy and Risk of Congenital Anomalies" analyzed the incidence of congenital birth defects among 16,350 and 16,088 live-born infants in Tdap exposed and unexposed live-births. The authors concluded that in eight body systems (eye, ear/face/neck, respiratory, upper GI tract, genitals, kidneys, and musculoskeletal system), there was a 17-100%+ greater chance of congenital malformation after vaccination.

Despite the concerning correlation between congenital defects and vaccinations, the study authors conclude that the vaccine is safe for pregnant women.

Conclusion: Tdap

The two FDA-approved Tdap vaccines are Adacel® and Boostrix®. According to the manufacturer's package insert for each, safety and effectiveness have not been established in pregnant women.[48,49] The available evidence suggests children exposed to Tdap during pregnancy may not have adequate protection against pertussis infection and may have a higher risk of congenital abnormalities. Fetal safety and efficacy have not been established.

RSV Vaccine

On September 22, 2023, the CDC's Advisory Committee on Immunization Practices recommended pregnant women between thirty-two and thirty-six weeks get vaccinated against the respiratory syncytial virus (RSV) with the recently FDA-approved Abrysvo®.[50] The CDC stated that all infants should be protected against RSV using Pfizer's Abrysvo®, either in utero or shortly after birth.

The CDC further noted that in clinical trials among pregnant women at twenty-four to twenty-six weeks, there were more preterm births observed among the RSV vaccine recipients than the unexposed. Other notable occurrences were a higher rate of preeclampsia, lower birth weight, and jaundice in the pregnant RSV-vaccinated women.[51] Despite these observations, the CDC promotes the vaccine in the last trimester of pregnancy.

What is RSV?

According to the CDC, RSV (respiratory syncytial virus) is a common respiratory virus that usually causes mild, cold-like symptoms that last for between one to two weeks.[52] RSV is the most common cause of lower respiratory tract infections in young children and adults. For the vast majority of people, RSV infection is like a cold. Accordingly, true prevalence is relatively unknown as the only people who are tested for it are those who are severely ill or in the hospital.[53]

Informed Consent?

Reported rising numbers of RSV infections and hospitalizations prompted major drug manufacturers to quickly develop vaccines.[54] In the drive to develop an RSV vaccine for pregnant women, two companies jumped on board: GlaxoSmithKline (GSK) and Pfizer. In early 2022, both were working on RSV-F protein vaccines to inoculate pregnant women to protect their babies.

Abruptly, GlaxoSmithKline halted their phase three trial upon observing a higher incidence of preterm deliveries in RSV-vaccinated pregnancies compared with the placebo group.[55] According to the FDA, the researchers recorded nearly a 40% increase in preterm births in the vaccine arm of the study.[56]

Pfizer continued with their trial but chose to withhold the GSK trial information from their pregnant study participants, which raised concerns over the completeness of informed consent.[57] Accordingly, the BMJ (*British Medical Journal*) investigated Pfizer's RSV vaccine clinical trial and the failure to share this information with the pregnant women.[58]

In their investigation, BMJ examined trial consent forms that stated the vaccine was "risk-free" for the baby. The BMJ also contacted governmental health authorities and trial investigators in the eighteen countries where trials were being conducted globally, asking if informed consent was provided. No one replied.

Preterm Births, Jaundice, Low Birth Weight, and Preeclampsia

Like the GSK clinical trial, more preterm births were observed among those vaccinated than those who received the placebo in Pfizer's Abrysvo trial.

The FDA labeled the potential risk as a warning and approved the vaccine for use in pregnant women at 32-36 weeks, citing a need to avoid the potential risks associated with a preterm birth before 32 weeks.[59] The World Health Organization and current studies, however, note that preterm births *less than 37 weeks of age* are the leading cause of neonatal morbidity and mortality globally.[60,61]

The CDC reported that the Pfizer trial found infants born to vaccinated mothers were more likely to have a low birth weight and neonatal jaundice. Low-birth weight babies are twenty times more likely to develop complications and die in comparison to normal weight babies.[62] Severe jaundice in newborns can cause brain damage, cerebral palsy, and hearing loss.[63]

Hypertension and preeclampsia occurred more frequently in vaccinated pregnant women than in those who were unvaccinated. Preeclampsia increases a woman's risk for organ damage to the kidneys, liver, and brain.[64] This hypertensive disorder can also increase the risk for developing life-threatening complications during birth, such as placenta separation and hemorrhage.[65]

Preeclampsia can progress to eclampsia, uncontrollable seizures that, when left untreated, can cause the death of both the mother and baby. Women who survive preeclampsia have reduced life expectancy and an increased risk of cardiovascular disease, diabetes, and stroke.[66] Babies born from preeclamptic pregnancies have increased risks of preterm births, perinatal death, and neurodevelopmental delay.[67]

Elevated risk of low birth weight and neonatal death in babies born to RSV-vaccinated mothers was confirmed in a separate study on a vaccine similar to Abrysvo™, which was approved by the FDA in 2023 to protect infants against RSV. Published in March 2024 in the *New England Journal of Medicine,* the study of more than 5000 women across 24 countries found a 37% increased risk of low birth weight and more than a doubling of neonatal deaths, although the latter result did not achieve statistical significance.[68] In light of these safety concerns, the clinical trial was stopped early due to the increased risk of preterm births.

Conclusion: RSV

In 2023, the CDC recommended that all pregnant women vaccinate with Pfizer's Abrysvo® RSV-vaccine to protect their unborn babies from the common respiratory virus. In their Morbidity and Mortality Weekly Report, the CDC informed the public that the pregnant women who received the vaccine experienced higher rates of preterm births and preeclampsia.[69] The report also stated that infants of vaccinated mothers had higher rates of jaundice and low birth weights. The ACIP (Advisory Committee on Immunization Practices) concluded that the benefits of the vaccine at thirty-two to thirty-six weeks' gestation outweighed these "potential" risks, and the FDA subsequently granted approval. The FDA should reconsider its approval.

CHAPTER 20

State Vaccine Requirements and Exemptions

Making Decisions Based on Risk/Benefit Analysis

Understanding the risk/benefit analysis of a given vaccine is the best approach when deciding whether and when to vaccinate a child. Not all vaccines are appropriate for all children. The ability to choose, however, has been heavily impacted by state school vaccine mandates.

States favor the benefit side of the risk/benefit equation by tying vaccination to public and even private education. The requirements are highly coercive and weigh heavily on the minds of many parents. The state effectively makes the choice for you, often substituting political choices in the name of the public good for informed choices made by parents, caregivers, and providers.

Political choices are always affected by the golden rule: those who have the gold, rule. Pharmaceutical and health products companies spent a record $372 million in 2022 lobbying Congress and federal agencies, outspending every other industry.[1] It was money well spent if the goal involved adding new vaccines to the Childhood Immunization Schedule.

Once on the schedule, vaccines never come off and are guaranteed to be insured or covered by the Vaccines for Children program.[2] Being added to the list is an annuity manufacturers have come to rely on.

Vaccination Exemptions

Although the CDC determines which vaccines will be on the Childhood Immunization Schedule, it is up to the states to determine vaccine requirements for school attendance. Further, each state establishes requirements for vaccine exemptions, which has resulted in a patchwork of requirements and exemptions across the fifty states.

There are three types of exemptions: medical, religious, and personal belief.

Medical exemptions usually entail physician documentation stating which vaccines can be omitted. Some states require medical justification for each exemption. In many states, an exemption can be revoked in the event of a disease outbreak.

Religious exemptions are based on the right of free exercise of religious beliefs. Required documentation requesting exemption is highly variable from state to state. As with medical exemptions, religious exemptions may be overridden in several states in the event of a disease outbreak.

Personal belief is just that: a parent or parents may hold a personal belief about vaccines that precludes their use. Documentation requirements are highly variable from state to state. As with medical and religious exemptions, personal belief exemptions may be overridden in several states in the event of a disease outbreak.

50-State Table of Exemptions

Links to each state's vaccine and exemptions requirements can be found via the QR code.

National Vaccine Information Center—State Vaccine Laws and Exemptions.

CHAPTER 21

Five Questions to Ask Your Pediatrician (or Other Vaccine Provider)

"What must not be, cannot be."
—Wolfgang Ehrengut, MD, German pediatrician, immunologist, and Professor of Vaccinology

Assumptions Underlying the Paradox of Unavoidably Unsafe

The concept of Unavoidably Unsafe was used to justify the potential risks of vaccines and absolve manufacturers of liability. It was predicated on four broad assumptions:

1. Vaccines are rigorously tested for safety and efficacy.
2. Risks of vaccines are offset by individual and societal benefits.
3. Learned intermediaries such as pediatricians or family physicians are capable of explaining the risks and benefits of vaccines to patients and their caregivers.[1]
4. Manufacturers will disclose all known risks of the vaccine to enable informed consent.

Unfortunately, adherence to these assumptions is the exception in relation to childhood vaccines.

Disclosure and Informed Consent Have Become Watered Down

Disclosure expectations were made clear in the 1985 National Research Council report to Congress that served as the basis for the 1986 National Child Vaccine Injury Act (NCVIA). The Council stated:

> [A] manufacturer will be liable if he markets a drug or vaccine with known risks and fails to warn of them, and it can be shown that the recipient would not have taken the drug or vaccine had he known of the risks.[2]

Unfortunately, this critical component of informed consent has been practiced more in the breach than in compliance.

For example, the CDC's Vaccine Information Statements (VIS) have been repeatedly watered down in substance to the point where the disclosures are so truncated that they are practically meaningless.

The original 1986 law required a VIS to include "the contraindications to (and bases for delay of) the administration of the vaccine," and "characteristics of recipients of the vaccine who may be at significantly higher risk of major adverse reaction to the vaccine than the general population."[3]

The 1993 amendment to the NCVIA was radical, trimming the existing ten guidelines for disclosure down to four. In the process, they removed the two examples above and other items like "early warning signs or symptoms . . . as possible precursors [of] major adverse reactions" and "symptoms or reactions to the vaccine which . . . should be brought to the immediate attention of a healthcare provider." By stripping down the information, they reduced the viability of informed consent.

Now, the following four items govern the NICIA policy without any practical definition of what is meant:[4]

1. A concise description of the benefits of the vaccine.
2. A concise description of the risks associated with the vaccine.
3. A statement of the availability of the National Vaccine Injury Program.
4. Such other relevant information that may be determined by the Secretary.

VIS is a Poor Substitute for Full Disclosure

By way of example, the Multi Pediatric Vaccines VIS includes summaries of five vaccines, including DTaP, Hib, Hep B, PCV, and Polio. (See details via QR code)

At best, the VIS skims the surface of these vaccines and certainly does not meet the original intent of disclosure outlined in the 1986 NCVIA. Compare the Multi Pediatric Vaccines VIS with the package insert with any of the five vaccines and superficiality of the VIS becomes apparent.

Here, for example, is the package insert for one of the DTaP vaccines:

Here, a package insert for a PCV vaccine:

Take a look at the Contents near the beginning of the form. All package inserts are structured in the same way and include:

FULL PRESCRIBING INFORMATION:

1. INDICATIONS AND USAGE [What the vaccine prevents or treats]
2. DOSAGE AND ADMINISTRATION [How much and how is it given]
3. DOSAGE FORMS AND STRENGTHS [Self-explanatory]
4. CONTRAINDICATIONS [Who should not get the vaccine]
5. WARNINGS AND PRECAUTIONS [Known side effects]
6. ADVERSE REACTIONS [What adverse reactions have been reported]
7. DRUG INTERACTIONS [Drugs that may interfere or accentuate activity]
8. USE IN SPECIFIC POPULATIONS [Who it is for]
9. DRUG ABUSE AND DEPENDENCY [Omitted for vaccines]
10. OVERDOSAGE [Omitted for vaccines]
11. DESCRIPTION [All the ingredients including excipients—if it contains aluminum compounds they will be listed here]
12. CLINICAL PHARMACOLOGY [Mechanism of Action]
13. NONCLINICAL TOXICOLOGY [Whether tested for Carcinogenesis, Mutagenesis, or Impairment of Fertility]
14. CLINICAL STUDIES [The basis for claims of effectiveness]
15. REFERENCES [Research citations]
16. HOW SUPPLIED/STORAGE AND HANDLING
17. PATIENT COUNSELING INFORMATION

Informed Consent

Few consumers are able to interpret such details, but the VIS as currently constructed is a poor substitute. Vaccine providers must be thoroughly familiar with package-insert level detail and be able to clearly explain it.

It is worth noting that vaccines authorized under Emergency Use Authorization have a blank package insert. Every pediatric COVID-19 mRNA vaccine marketed under an EUA in the US for children under twelve was exempt from package insert-level disclosure, making full informed consent impossible. Instead, vaccines issued under an EUA have a VIS and an EUA fact sheet, neither of which contain the full disclosure provided by a package insert.[5]

Elements of Informed Consent

Informed consent to medical treatment is fundamental in both ethics and law. Parents and guardians have the right to receive information and ask questions about recommended vaccines so that they can make informed decisions on behalf of minors. Consent should not be presumed by providers or coerced. Threats to discontinue care if vaccination is declined are unethical and raise legal issues of patient abandonment.

The nature of a truly informed consent is perhaps best expressed in the Belmont Report's "Ethical Principles and Guidelines for the Protection of Human Subjects of Research."[6] The report was prepared in response to the 1974 Research Act that charged a Commission for Protection of Human Subjects to identify basic ethical principles of informed consent. The Commission provided a valuable framework to consider noting there was "widespread agreement that the consent process [has] three elements: information, comprehension and voluntariness."[7]

Although the Belmont Report discussed informed consent for research subjects in particular, it serves as sound guidance for vaccine consent as well. Informed consent for vaccines should include disclosure of information regarding risks and benefits to the child, confirmation the parent or guardian understands the information, and affirmation that consent was not the result of a threat to withhold care.

This is particularly important in the case of COVID-19 mRNA vaccines authorized under an EUA as they are exempt from many of the clinical trial, manufacturing, and informed consent requirements demanded of other vaccines and biologics. In effect, children under twelve who are vaccinated become test subjects for an experimental therapy without parental or guardian informed consent.

Vaccine Consent Forms

Many versions of a vaccine consent form are available.[8,9,10] Most are quite thorough in terms of past medical history, previous immunizations, allergies and so forth and may even ask if the parent has reviewed the VIS relevant to a particular vaccine.

Provided the child has no medical contraindication to be vaccinated, they all presume vaccination will proceed. In other words, they are simply *consent* forms not *informed consent* forms. None of them address core issues such as how likely your child is to get the disease or the availability/effectiveness of treatments for the disease targeted by the vaccine. Notably, the VIS does **not** include information about alternative vaccine schedules or delaying the shot.

Here They Are: Five Questions to Ask Before Letting Someone Vaccinate Your Child

In light of the inadequacy of clinical trials for many pediatric vaccines, the regulatory exemptions vaccines are granted compared with other biologicals and drugs, and the insufficiency of the CDC's Vaccine Information Statements, it is essential for your pediatrician or other vaccine provider to serve as your learned advocate.

In addition to the standard information obtained in most consent forms, the following five questions offer the best opportunity to inform a decision about vaccinating a child.

1. **How likely is my child to get the disease?**
    a. Is the disease common?
    b. Can it be avoided or minimized in other ways?
    c. What if my child has already contracted the disease?
2. **Is my child considered to be at high risk of severe illness?**
    a. Does my child have any special risk factors?
    b. What measures can be taken to mitigate my child's risk or risk to others without vaccination?
    c. If my child is at low risk, can I defer the scheduled vaccines until a later date?
3. **Are treatments available if my child contracts the disease?**
    a. What early interventions should we consider?
    b. Are there repurposed drugs (prescription medications not approved for this indication but are in common use) available for treatment?
    c. Are there over-the-counter drugs or supplements that can improve my child's outcome?
4. **Is there a test to show if my child has immunity from a previous infection?**
    a. What blood or other tests will indicate whether my child has natural immunity?
    b. If my child has natural immunity, does he/she still need a vaccination? If so, why?
5. **Have you reviewed the package insert for the vaccine(s) and can you explain it to me?**
    a. Was vaccine effectiveness determined by antibody studies or by clinical safety and outcome trials? If antibody studies, how confident are you that they translate into clinical effectiveness?
    b. What was the Absolute Risk Reduction for a child who receives the vaccine and how does that compare with the reported Relative Risk Reduction?
    c. Do you consider any vaccine excipients (ingredients) to be toxic—what excipients are included and is there any aluminum?
    d. What placebo was used in the placebo control group or groups? If it was a biologically active ingredient like aluminum, how certain are you about its vaccine safety?
    e. What are the three most frequent serious adverse events I should be aware of?

It is expected that most pediatricians and other vaccine providers will readily engage in such dialogue. They are overwhelmingly committed to their patients and want to provide the best care. Some physicians may possess a negative bias against vaccine injury. Vaccine benefits have been strongly inculcated into physicians throughout their training. That can lead to a mindset that vaccine injury must not be true because physicians are at a loss about what to do if it is true.

As Dr. Ehrengut said, "What must not be, cannot be."[11]

It is also entirely possible that physicians' work schedules preclude being up to date on the latest vaccine information. Unless parents and other caregivers press for this information, a full set of on-schedule vaccinations will proceed without question.

But physicians are under increasing pressure to conform. Unfortunately, trusted medical associations have become more politically active in an effort to suppress vaccine "misinformation" deemed contrary to FDA and CDC positions.

The American Academy of Pediatrics and the American Academy of Family Physicians support the government's efforts to require social media companies to censor medical opinions at their direction. These organizations have filed a legal brief in support of the government's position in the Missouri v Biden free speech case being heard by the Supreme Court.[12]

In their brief, the medical societies argue that the government has a compelling interest in combating vaccine misinformation because it can decrease vaccine uptake, diminish vaccines' ability to control disease, and reduce the number of lives saved.[13]

A ruling in support of the government would effectively prevent many of the arguments made in this book from being disseminated through social media. In fact, it would be even more difficult to promote the book as a whole, given that its purpose is to raise legitimate scientific issues about the risks and benefits of childhood vaccines so parents can be better informed advocates for their children.

One may disagree with any or all of the points made in this book, but it should be clear from the evidence presented that the FDA and CDC have their thumbs on the benefits side of the vaccine scale. Moreover, the government should never be in the position to decide what is "true" and what is "misinformation" and then subsequently suppress any speech with which it disagrees. Censorship is never the way to resolve controversy; only more information and discourse can hope to resolve differences of opinion.

Any vaccine provider unwilling to have a candid discussion with you about vaccines may simply be too busy or has submitted to the decrees of the CDC and professional organizations. If that is the case, seek out a provider who will take the time to engage in a reasoned discussion about vaccines.

Sadly, the American Academy of Pediatrics has responded in counterproductive fashion to increasing skepticism by parents about the benefits versus risks of vaccines.

In 2005, AAP recommended that, "pediatricians should avoid discharging patients from their practice solely because a parent refuses to immunize his or her child."[14] AAP changed its policy in 2016 to one of intolerance, stating, "a pediatrician may consider dismissal of families who refuse vaccination as an acceptable option," albeit acknowledging they should respect the beliefs of the family in question.[15, 16] AAP does not explain how dismissing a family from a practice respects their beliefs nor has it demonstrated that refusal to provide care improves vaccine uptake.

Speak with other parents about their vaccine experience and share notes about providers who are willing to engage on this important topic.

CHAPTER 22

Conclusion

The goal of childhood vaccination should not be to eliminate infection. It's simply not feasible to do so. Pathogens have infinite capacity to mutate and evade any conceived vaccination strategy.

Smallpox may be the exception that proves the rule: survivors were immune for life, there were no animal reservoirs, cases were isolated, and perhaps most importantly, the virus mutated slowly, enabling widespread immunity through global use of a stable vaccine.[1]

The rest of the viral kingdom has not been so compliant. For example, respiratory viruses have defied all efforts at control through vaccination. They rapidly mutate their way around immunity induced by vaccines. Influenza vaccines are practically obsolete before they hit the market, often failing to achieve a threshold of 50% efficacy and never for more than one season. There is even evidence that repeat influenza vaccination increases the risk of infection.

Forty years of effort and over $12 billion have failed to create an HIV vaccine.[2] Fortunately, effective antiviral therapies have filled the gap left by vaccine development failures.

Bacterial vaccines are similarly challenged. In 2000, pneumococcal vaccines started with seven covered bacterial strains, but declining vaccine effectiveness drove the addition of sixteen more strains in the intervening years. And yet, around seventy strains remain uncovered.

Perhaps more importantly, humans and germs have coexisted for thousands of generations. Exposure to viruses, bacteria, and other pathogens early in life helps young immune systems to mature, build a robust memory of threats, and learn how to modulate a proportional response to invaders.

Just Like Healthy Bones, Young Immune Systems Need to Be Stressed to Gain Strength

Childhood vaccination can interfere with normal immune development and compromise durable, lifelong natural immunity. Failure of the immune system to learn how to distinguish harmful organisms from self without overreaction can lead to autoimmune disorders. Many of the vaccines and excipients discussed in this book have been implicated in immune dysregulation.

The goal of vaccination should be to prepare for threats that either evade or overwhelm the immature immune system, using a technically stable vaccine platform that is safe and well-tested.

Appropriate, universal childhood vaccine targets exist . . . or have existed. They include diseases like smallpox, now extinct thanks to vaccination and other factors unique to the variola virus; polio, which can rapidly attack the nervous system prior to natural immune response; hepatitis B, which can evade natural immunity to become a chronic and deadly infection; and tetanus, which is a toxin, not an infection.

Other examples include vaccination to prevent rubella and varicella infection during pregnancy, vital to prevent fetal abnormalities. But even here, the vaccines are only necessary if the mother has a low level of antibodies or was not infected during childhood (which confers lifelong immunity).

Risk-benefit analysis for PCV (pneumococcal) and Hib (H. influenza) vaccines present a conundrum. As discussed in previous chapters, each bacterial disease can cause devastating symptoms, which favors their use. On the other hand, each has safety risks and their immunity wanes following vaccination, largely due to emergence of resistant or replacement strains.

Then of course there are children with underlying illnesses, prematurity, immune suppression, chemotherapy, and so forth, who need vaccines to protect them from common diseases. Discussion of vaccination for this vulnerable group is beyond the scope of this book.

Just Because Scientists Can, Doesn't Mean They Should

Creating new vaccines to chase after all manner of diseases that rarely cause serious illness or death in healthy children is rarely justified. Just because it is possible to do so, creating a new vaccine does not automatically serve children's best interests.

Even if a new vaccine based on novel technology has the potential for public benefit, it must be weighed against the risks. Where vaccines are concerned, there is never an absence of risk. The application of the mRNA vaccine platform to COVID-19 vaccines is a prime example of an enabling technology that came to market prematurely, the consequences of which are still being uncovered.

In fact, it can be argued that the general health of children has been in decline since passage of the 1986 National Childhood Vaccine Injury Act, with rising rates of asthma, ASD, and allergies. The public is beginning to take notice that the addition of each new vaccine to the Childhood Vaccine Schedule looks to be less in the public health interest and more like a lucrative protection racket for the manufacturers.

Even the Institute of Medicine acknowledged that most vaccine-related research ignores the addition of new vaccines in the context of the overall vaccine schedule:

> Most vaccine-related research focuses on the outcomes of single immunizations or combinations of vaccines administered at a single visit. Although each new vaccine is evaluated in the context of the overall immunization schedule that existed at the time of review of that vaccine, elements of the schedule are not evaluated once it is adjusted to accommodate a new vaccine. Thus, key elements of the entire schedule—the number, frequency, timing, order, and age at administration of vaccines—have not been systematically examined in research studies.[3]

The revolving door between the federal regulators and the vaccine manufacturers calls into question whose interests are being served by the FDA, CDC, and other federal agencies assigned to protect the public health and how aggressively they will pursue the many unanswered questions about vaccine safety.

Key Takeaways from This Book

Regulators

- The revolving door between the FDA, CDC, HHS, and Big Pharma has undermined trust in and the integrity of federal regulatory agencies who are chartered to protect the public health.
- The regulatory apparatus that is meant to protect the public from unsafe and ineffective vaccines is broken.
- The regulatory process has been watered down and rendered inadequate since the good intentions of the 1986 National Childhood Vaccine Injury Act (NCVIA).
- CDC altered the definition of a vaccine, lowering the standard for approval.
- The FDA does not hold vaccines to the same safety, clinical, or manufacturing standards as other biologics or drugs.
- Emergency Use Authorization of a vaccine can be triggered by mere declaration of a Public Health Emergency by the Secretary of HHS.
- Emergency Use Authorization relies on subjective and arbitrary vaccine authorization criteria that undermine patient protections.

Legislation

- The 1986 NCVIA provides blanket liability protection for vaccine manufacturers—the Act federalized the liabilities and privatized the profits.

- Congress should repeal liability protection from the 1986 NCVIA so that manufacturers remain incentivized to make safer vaccines.

Lack of Adequate Clinical Trials

- Childhood vaccines for children under twelve have never been subjected to randomized, placebo-controlled clinical trials, considered the gold standard for clinical studies.
- The FDA does not require randomized, placebo-controlled clinical trials prior to vaccine approval.
- Vaccine trials report effectiveness using Relative Risk Reduction (RRR) that can make vaccine efficacy look much more impressive than it is.
- Absolute Risk Reduction (ARR) may allow a more accurate assessment of vaccine efficacy for any given child and should be part of any risk-benefit analysis.
- Childhood vaccines contain known toxins and powerful immune stimulators that have not been adequately tested for safety.
- American children receive more vaccines by twelve months, the period of greatest developmental vulnerability, than that of any other country.
- The health of American children has declined since the 1986 NCVIA in terms of allergies, asthma, autism spectrum disorder and obesity.

Stop Blaming the Unvaccinated

- Stop blaming the unvaccinated.
- Children should not have to bear the risk of vaccination in order to protect others through herd immunity if they risk harm from vaccines or aren't themselves at high risk.
- Vaccines either work or they don't work—isolate as needed and protect the vulnerable.
- Children should not be the first line of defense for at-risk adults.

Natural Immunity is Durable and Effective

- Childhood infections build effective immune systems that have a long memory for past pathogens, anticipate mutations in those pathogens, and respond proportionately to infection without overreacting.
- Immunizations can interfere with building of natural immunity.
- The CDC acknowledges that previous infection with common childhood diseases such as chickenpox, measles, mumps and rubella precludes the need for vaccination due to natural immunity.
- The majority of people born before 1957 are likely to have been infected naturally and therefore are presumed to be protected against measles, mumps, and rubella.

- Support for developing young immune systems includes fresh air, sunshine, regular activity, socialization, stimulation of the mind, and a diet low in sweets and carbohydrates.

Herd Immunity

- Vaccines can never completely replace natural immunity.
- Vaccines can contribute to herd immunity, but true herd immunity requires healthy immune systems across a broad population.
- Vaccines have the potential to compromise immune responses to future variants by training the immune system to look only for a single or limited set of antigens, as is the case with COVID-19 mRNA vaccines and the Spike protein.
- An ever-growing constellation of vaccines administered to children may ultimately undermine efforts to create herd immunity.

What Is Not Taught in Medical School

Medical schools assert they devote considerable time to vaccine education. The reality is that doctors in training generally do not receive in-depth training about vaccines regarding the following essentials:

- Manufacturing processes—differentiating between traditional culture media techniques, recombinant production, and custom mRNA synthesis technologies.
- Implications of modified mRNA, self-amplifying mRNA, and lipid nanoparticle transport mechanisms on vaccine distribution, toxicity, and degradation, immune dysregulation, hypersensitivity disorders, and autoimmunity.
- Emergency Use Authorization versus Biologics License Application (BLA) Approval process requirements and implications for vaccine safety testing and effectiveness.
- Manufacturer protection provisions of the 1986 National Childhood Vaccine Injury Act.
- Vaccine Approval process as distinct from other biologics and drugs, including vaccine clinical testing requirements.
- How to read and interpret a vaccine package insert for patients.
- The distinction between a package insert, a Vaccine Information Statement (VIS), and an EUA Fact Sheet.
- Calculation of vaccine absolute versus relative risk reduction and how to interpret the results for patients.
- Risks of biologically active excipients, and toxicity of aluminum compounds in particular.
- Post-marketing passive and active surveillance systems.

- Submission of a VAERS report.
- Query and interpretation of the VAERS database.

Difficult for Providers to Keep Up, Pressure to Conform

- Many vaccine providers rely on the CDC and their professional associations for guidance about vaccination due to their own inability to keep up with developments in the field.
- Many professional organizations receive financial compensation from government organizations in order to promote vaccines.
- The American Academy of Pediatrics and the American Academy of Family Medicine have advocated for government censorship of vaccine "misinformation," depriving doctors and families or alternative sources of information and points of view.
- Many vaccine providers work for a larger group or health system that determines vaccination protocols on their behalf or exerts peer pressure to conform to the accepted schedule.
- Some physicians may have negative vaccine bias against the idea of vaccine injury.

Informed Consent

- Informed consent for childhood vaccination has devolved into a pro forma, cursory exercise.
- Informed consent has become a consent form.
- CDC Vaccine Information Statements lack specificity of information about safety and efficacy.
- Caregivers should request vaccine providers to review with them the vaccine package insert.
- Consent should not be presumed or coerced by providers.
- Threats to discontinue care if vaccination is declined are unethical and raise legal issues of patient abandonment.
- Fear should never be a factor when deciding to grant consent for treatment.

Risk-Benefit Assessments

Every child deserves an individual risk-benefit assessment for each vaccine prior to administration.

- Few providers are capable of such a detailed assessment, whether due to time restriction, lack of knowledge or health system mandates.
- Ask vaccine providers to provide each vaccine's Relative Risk Reduction compared with its Absolute Risk Reduction in order to better understand the vaccine's potential benefit for a child (this book provides several examples).

- In the face of uncertain benefit, consideration may be given to delaying vaccines in healthy children until at least after the first twelve months, and preferably two years, if elimination is not medically indicated or practical.

mRNA Vaccines Pose Special Risks

- mRNA vaccines should never be given to children or pregnant women.
- mRNA is actually modified RNA, which resists breakdown by natural enzymes and immune response.
- Once injected, modRNA continues making toxic and inflammatory Spike proteins for days to months after injection.
- Lipid nanoparticles (LNPs) are toxic themselves and transport the modRNA throughout the body, crossing the blood-brain barrier and entering the reproductive organs.
- The synthetic component of modRNA causes frameshifting or misreading of the RNA code inside the cells of the vaccinated, leading to production of potentially dangerous junk proteins that can elicit an inflammatory response.
- modRNA uses manufacturing techniques that have been shown to contaminate vaccine production with excessive amounts of foreign DNA.
- Foreign DNA left over from the manufacturing process is carried into cells by the LNPs.
- The risk of foreign DNA entering into human cells is not zero.

Vaccines and Autism, SIDS

- Vaccines as a cause of autism or SIDS has been neither proven nor disproven.
- Only one vaccine has been studied as a cause of autism—MMR.
- Only one excipient has been studied as a cause of autism—Thimerosal.

Vaccines and Pregnancy

- Vaccines recommended during pregnancy have not been proven either safe or effective.
- Critical safety data regarding COVID-19 mRNA released in 2023 (by federal court order) provides evidence of serious risk to both mothers and their babies.

HPV Vaccine

- HPV vaccine has not been proven either safe or effective.
- HPV vaccine benefits have been significantly overstated and misrepresented as reducing the incidence of cervical cancer.

School Vaccine Requirements and Exemptions

- School vaccine requirements have become the enforcement arm for the Childhood Vaccine Schedule.
- Exemptions (philosophical, religious, or medical) from school vaccine requirements vary widely by state, are themselves coercive, and should be understood by parents, guardians and clinicians as part of any decision to vaccinate a child (see Chapter 20, State Vaccine Requirements and Exemptions).

Pharmaceutical Companies and Politics

- Vaccine compliance has evolved to become as much a political tool as an informed medical decision.
- The pharmaceutical lobby has enormous influence over the political and regulatory process through lobbying and a wide-open revolving door.
- COVID-19 vaccine rapid authorization, compliance requirements and addition to the Childhood Immunization Schedule is a signal example of the triumph of political influence over science.
- Educating and organizing with other concerned parents and caregivers will be the only way to exert counterpressure and restore integrity to the vaccine juggernaut.

Become an Informed Advocate

Use this book to become an informed advocate for your child or the child under your care. Do not accept the status quo as being in your child's best interest.

Question and engage vaccine providers to make the best decision about childhood vaccination. And . . . share this book with others to keep the discussion alive.

Recommended resources for ongoing information about vaccines include the World Council for Health, Physicians for Informed Consent, and National Vaccine Information Center, which can be found via the QR codes below:

The World Council for Health

Physicians for Informed Consent

National Vaccine Information Center

Endnotes

Prologue

1 Kanter, Genevieve P., and Daniel Carpenter. "The Revolving Door in Health Care Regulation." *Health Affairs* 42, no. 9 (September 1, 2023): 1298–1303. https://doi.org/10.1377/hlthaff.2023.00418.

2 Federal Register. "Removal of Certain Time of Inspection and Duties of Inspector Regulations for Biological Products; Companion to Direct Final Rule." January 26, 2018. https://www.federalregister.gov/documents/2018/01/26/2018-01467/removal-of-certain-time-of-inspection-and-duties-of-inspector-regulations-for-biological-products.

3 Ibid.

4 Federal Register. "Removal of Certain Time of Inspection and Duties of Inspector Regulations for Biological Products." April 2, 2019. https://www.federalregister.gov/documents/2019/04/02/2019-06187/removal-of-certain-time-of-inspection-and-duties-of-inspector-regulations-for-biological-products.

5 Ibid.

6 Watt, Katherine. "Legalized FDA Non-Regulation of Biological Products Effective May 2, 2019, by Federal Register Final Rule, Signed by Then-FDA Commissioner Scott Gottlieb." Bailiwick News (blog), December 19, 2023. https://bailiwicknews.substack.com/p/legalized-fda-non-regulation-of-biological?r=o3im2&utm_campaign=post&utm_medium=web.

7 Peebles, Angelica. "Outgoing FDA Chief Scott Gottlieb Gets Personal about Leaving 'the Best Job' He's Ever Had." CNBC, April 2, 2019. https://www.cnbc.com/2019/03/31/outgoing-fda-chief-gottlieb-gets-personal-about-leaving-the-best-job.html.

8 Salary.com. "PFIZER INC Board Member Scott Gottlieb, M.D." https://www.salary.com/research/executive-compensation/scott-gottlieb-m-d-board-member-of-pfizer-inc.

9 Office of the Commissioner. "FDA Approves First COVID-19 Vaccine." U.S. Food And Drug Administration, August 23, 2021. https://www.fda.gov/news-events/press-announcements/fda-approves-first-covid-19-vaccine.

10 Silver, Kate. "Shot of a Lifetime: How Two Pfizer Manufacturing Plants Upscaled to Produce the COVID-19 Vaccine in Record Time | Pfizer." Accessed January 20, 2024. https://www.pfizer.com/news/articles/shot_of_a_lifetime_how_two_pfizer_manufacturing_plants_upscaled_to_produce_the_covid_19_vaccine_in_record_time.

11 Pfizer 2022 Annual Report. "Pfizer's Financial Performance in 2022." Accessed January 20, 2024. https://www.pfizer.com/sites/default/files/investors/financial_reports/annual_reports/2022/performance/.

12 Tanne, Janice Hopkins. "Pfizer Pays Record Fine for Off-Label Promotion of Four Drugs." *BMJ* 339 (2009): b3657. doi: 10.1136/bmj.b3657.

13 "Official Mission/Function Statement." Centers for Disease Control and Prevention. January 24, 2023. https://www.cdc.gov/about/pdf/organization/iod-mission-statement.pdf.Merck.com.

14 "Merck Announces Fourth-Quarter and Full-Year 2022 Financial Results." January 20, 2024. https://www.merck.com/news/merck-announces-fourth-quarter-and-full-year-2022-financial-results/.

15 Foley, Katherine Ellen. "Trust Issues Deepen as Yet Another FDA Commissioner Joins the Pharmaceutical Industry." *Quartz*, July 21, 2022. https://qz.com/1656529/yet-another-fda-commissioner-joins-the-pharmaceutical-industry.

16 Kanter, Genevieve P., and Daniel Carpenter. "The Revolving Door in Health Care Regulation." *Health Affairs* 42, no. 9 (September 1, 2023): 1298–1303. https://doi.org/10.1377/hlthaff.2023.00418.

Chapter 1

1 Tapper, Ben (@DrBenTapper1). "The thing that bugs me is that the people think the FDA is protecting them. It isn't." Twitter, September 17, 2023. https://twitter.com/drbentapper1/status/1703570723925614818?s=66&t=cDmaiTY_x7iU6MrD2vS9mQ.

2 "The Epidemic Of Poliomyelitis In New York, 1916." *The British Medical Journal* 2, no. 2950 (1917): 51–51. http://www.jstor.org/stable/20307769.

3 *File:The Seattle Star July 05 1916 Polio Epidemic .Jpg—Wikimedia Commons*. July 5, 1916. https://commons.wikimedia.org/w/index.php?curid=107263332.

4 The Regents of the University of Michigan. "1955 Polio Vaccine Trial Announcement." https://sph.umich.edu/polio/.

5 Lien, Gemma, and David L. Heymann. "The Problems with Polio: Toward Eradication." *Infectious Diseases and Therapy* 2, no. 2 (September 17, 2013): 167–74. https://www.ncbi.nlm.nih.gov/pmc/articles/PMC4108111/.

6 National Academies Press (US). "Polio Vaccines." Adverse Events Associated With Childhood Vaccines—NCBI Bookshelf, 1994. https://www.ncbi.nlm.nih.gov/books/NBK236293/.

7 Offit, Paul A. *The Cutter Incident: How America's First Polio Vaccine Led to the Growing Vaccine Crisis*, Yale University Press, 2005, 100–33.

8 "Influenza Historic Timeline 1930 and Beyond." Centers for Disease Control and Prevention, January 30, 2019. https://archive.cdc.gov/#/details?url=https://www.cdc.gov/flu/pandemic-resources/pandemic-timeline-1930-and-beyond.htm.

9 Ibid.

10 "Diphtheria-Tetanus-Pertussis Vaccine Shortage—United States." Centers for Disease Control and Prevention. *Morbidity and Mortality Weekly Report* 33, no.

49, (December 1984): 695–96. https://www.cdc.gov/mmwr/preview/mmwrhtml/00000452.htm.

11 National Research Council (US) Division of Health Promotion and Disease Prevention, *Vaccine Supply and Innovation.* Washington DC: National Academies Press; 1985. https://www.ncbi.nlm.nih.gov/books/NBK216810/.

12 Ibid.

13 National Academies Press (US). "Vaccine Injury Compensation and Liability Remedies." Vaccine Supply and Innovation—NCBI Bookshelf, 1985. https://www.ncbi.nlm.nih.gov/books/NBK216805/.

14 Nicholson, Christie. "What Is an Unavoidably Unsafe Product?" FindLaw, November 13, 2023. https://www.findlaw.com/injury/product-liability/what-is-an-unavoidably-unsafe-product.html.

15 National Academies Press (US). "Liability for the Production and Sale of Vaccines." Vaccine Supply and Innovation—NCBI Bookshelf, 1985. https://www.ncbi.nlm.nih.gov/books/NBK216813/#rrr00125.

16 Justia Law. "Bruesewitz v. Wyeth LLC, 562 U.S. 223 (2011)." Accessed January 20, 2024. https://supreme.justia.com/cases/federal/us/562/223/.

17 National Academies Press (US). "Vaccine Injury Compensation and Liability Remedies." Vaccine Supply and Innovation—NCBI Bookshelf, 1985. https://www.ncbi.nlm.nih.gov/books/NBK216805/.

18 National Academies Press (US). "Liability for the Production and Sale of Vaccines." Vaccine Supply and Innovation—NCBI Bookshelf, 1985. https://www.ncbi.nlm.nih.gov/books/NBK216813/.

19 "Vaccine Information Statement | Current VISS | CDC." Centers for Disease Control and Prevention. December 7, 2023. https://www.cdc.gov/vaccines/hcp/vis/current-vis.html.

20 "HHS Announces $22 Billion in Funding to Support Expanded Testing, Vaccination Distribution." Centers for Disease Control and Prevention. January 7, 2021. https://archive.cdc.gov/#/details?url=https://www.cdc.gov/media/releases/2021/p0107-covid-19-funding.html.

21 Miller, A. "CDC to Reduce Funding for States' Child Vaccination Programs." *Scientific American.* July 7, 2023. https://www.scientificamerican.com/article/cdc-to-reduce-funding-for-states-child-vaccination-programs/.

22 "Vaccine Schedule for Children 6 Years or Younger | CDC." Centers for Disease Control and Prevention. Accessed January 20, 2024. https://www.cdc.gov/vaccines/schedules/easy-to-read/child-easyread.html.

23 Miller, Neil Z., and Gary S. Goldman. "Infant Mortality Rates Regressed Against Number of Vaccine Doses Routinely Given: Is There a Biochemical or Synergistic Toxicity?" *Human & Experimental Toxicology* 30, no. 9 (May 4, 2011): 1420–28. https://www.ncbi.nlm.nih.gov/pmc/articles/PMC3170075/.

24 Justia Law. "Bruesewitz v. Wyeth LLC, 562 U.S. 223 (2011)." Accessed January 20, 2024. https://supreme.justia.com/cases/federal/us/562/223/.

25 Phillips, Aleks. "Pfizer Accused of 'Obscene' COVID Profits after Posting Record Revenues." *Newsweek*, February 2, 2023. https://www.newsweek.com/pfizer-obscene-covid-pandemic-profits-record-revenues-1778513.

Chapter 2

1 Angell, Marcia. "Big Pharma, Bad Medicine." *Boston Review*. May 1, 2010. https://www.bostonreview.net/forum/angell-big-pharma-bad-medicine/.

2 U.S. Food and Drug Administration. "CFR—Code of Federal Regulations Title 21." October 17, 2023. https://www.accessdata.fda.gov/scripts/cdrh/cfdocs/cfcfr/CFRSearch.cfm?fr=600.3.

3 Ibid.

4 World Council for Health. "A Common-Sense Approach to Childhood Vaccines Is Now Needed." *World Council for Health*, September 5, 2023. https://worldcouncilforhealth.org/news/statements/childhood-vaccines/.

5 "Immunization: The Basics." Centers of Disease Control and Prevention. Feb 24, 2011. https://web.archive.org/web/20120307022707/http://www.cdc.gov/vaccines/vac-gen/imz-basics.htm.

6 "Immunization: The Basics." Centers for Disease Control and Prevention. May 16, 2018. https://web.archive.org/web/20210826113846/https://www.cdc.gov/vaccines/vac-gen/imz-basics.htm.

7 "Immunization: The Basics." Centers for Disease Control and Prevention. September 1, 2021. https://www.cdc.gov/vaccines/vac-gen/imz-basics.htm.

8 "Adjuvants and Vaccines | Vaccine Safety | CDC." Centers for Disease Control and Prevention. September 27, 2002. https://www.cdc.gov/vaccinesafety/concerns/adjuvants.html.

9 Dowling, David J., and Levy Ofer. "Pediatric Vaccine Adjuvants." *The Pediatric Infectious Disease Journal* 34, no. 12 (December 1, 2015): 1395–98. https://www.ncbi.nlm.nih.gov/pmc/articles/PMC4931280/.

10 McKernan, Kevin, Yvonne Helbert, Liam T. Kane, and Stephen McLaughlin. 2023. "Sequencing of Bivalent Moderna and Pfizer Mrna Vaccines Reveals Nanogram to Microgram Quantities of Expression Vector Dsdna Per Dose." *OSF Preprints*. April 10. https://osf.io/b9t7m/.

11 Mold, Matthew, Emma Shardlow, and Christopher Exley. "Insight into the Cellular Fate and Toxicity of Aluminium Adjuvants Used in Clinically Approved Human Vaccinations." *Scientific Reports* 6, no. 1 (August 12, 2016). https://doi.org/10.1038/srep31578.

12 Ibid.

13 Goullé, J. P., and L. Grangeot-Keros. "Aluminum and Vaccines: Current State of Knowledge." *Médecine et Maladies Infectieuses* 50, no. 1 (2020): 16–21. https://www.sciencedirect.com/science/article/pii/S0399077X18308448.

14 Fulgenzi, Alessandro, Daniele Vietti, and Maria Elena Ferrero. "Aluminum Involvement in Neurotoxicity." *BioMed Research International* 2014 (2014): 1–5. https://doi.org/10.1155/2014/758323.

15 Tomljenovic, L., and C. A. Shaw. "Aluminum Vaccine Adjuvants: Are They Safe?" *Current Medicinal Chemistry* 18, no. 17 (2011): 2630–37. https://doi.org/10.2174/092986711795933740.

16 Mold, Matthew, Caroline Linhart, Johana Gómez-Ramírez, Andrés Villegas-Lanau, and Christopher Exley. "Aluminum and Amyloid-β in Familial Alzheimer's Disease." *Journal of Alzheimer's Disease* 73, no. 4 (2020): 1627–35. https://content.iospress.com/articles/journal-of-alzheimers-disease/jad191140.

17 Mold, Matthew, Dorcas Umar, Andrew King, and Christopher Exley. "Aluminum in Brain Tissue in Autism." *Journal of Trace Elements in Medicine and Biology* 46 (2018): 76–82. https://www.sciencedirect.com/science/article/pii/S0946672X17308763?via%3Dihub.

18 Exley, Christopher, and Elizabeth Clarkson. "Aluminium in Human Brain Tissue from Donors without Neurodegenerative Disease: A Comparison with Alzheimer's Disease, Multiple Sclerosis and Autism." *Scientific Reports* 10, no. 1 (2020). https://www.nature.com/articles/s41598-020-64734-6.

19 Wang, Liuyongwei, Linqiang Mei, Zhenle Zang, Yun Cai, Peiyan Jiang, Lianyu Zhou, Zhulin Du, et al. "Aluminum Hydroxide Exposure Induces Neurodevelopmental Impairment in HESC-Derived Cerebral Organoids." *Ecotoxicology and Environmental Safety* 256 (2023): 114863. https://doi.org/10.1016/j.ecoenv.2023.114863.

20 "Aluminum." WHO Food Additives Series 24. Accessed January 23, 2024. https://inchem.org/documents/jecfa/jecmono/v024je07.htm#.

21 "Adjuvants and Vaccines." Centers for Disease Control and Prevention, September 27, 2022https://www.cdc.gov/vaccinesafety/concerns/adjuvants.html.

22 Guimarães, Luísa Eça, Britain Baker, Carlo Perricone, and Yehuda Shoenfeld. "Vaccines, Adjuvants and Autoimmunity." Pharmacological Research 100 (2015): 190–209. https://doi.org/10.1016/j.phrs.2015.08.003.

23 "Incredibly Deceptive" HPV Vaccine Propaganda With Michael Baum + Mary Holland. Children's Health Defense, 2023. https://live.childrenshealthdefense.org/chd-tv/shows/good-morning-chd/incredibly-deceptive-hpv-vaccine-propaganda-with-michael-baum—mary-holland/?utm_source=luminate&utm_medium=email&utm_campaign=chdtv&utm_id=20231213.

24 "Vaccine Adjuvant." ScienceDirect. Accessed January 23, 2024. https://www.sciencedirect.com/topics/pharmacology-toxicology-and-pharmaceutical-science/vaccine-adjuvant.

25 Watad, Abdulla, Kassem Sharif, and Yehuda Shoenfeld. "The Asia Syndrome: Basic Concepts." *Mediterranean Journal of Rheumatology* 28, no. 2 (2017): 64–69. https://doi.org/10.31138/mjr.28.2.64.

26 Daley, Matthew F., Liza M. Reifler, Jason M. Glanz, Simon J. Hambidge, Darios Getahun, Stephanie A. Irving, James D. Nordin, et al. "Association between Aluminum Exposure from Vaccines before Age 24 Months and Persistent Asthma at Age 24 to 59 Months." *Academic Pediatrics* 23, no. 1 (2023): 37–46. https://doi.org/10.1016/j.acap.2022.08.006.

27 Linhart, Caroline, Sameerah Connor, Erin Softely, and Christopher Exley. "The Measurement and Full Statistical Analysis Including Bayesian Methods of the Aluminium Content of Infant Vaccines." *Journal of Trace Elements in Medicine and Biology* 66 (2011): 126762. https://doi.org/10.1016/j.jtemb.2021.126762.

28 Ibid.

29 Ibid.

30 Ibid.

31 "Vaccine Excipient Summary." Centers for Disease Control and Prevention, November 1, 2021. https://www.cdc.gov/vaccines/pubs/pinkbook/downloads/appendices/b/excipient-table-2.pdf.

32 "Vaccination Coverage for Selected Diseases by Age 24 Months, by Race and Hispanic Origin, Poverty Level, and Location of Residence: United States, Birth Years 2010–2016." Centers for Disease Control, 2020. https://www.cdc.gov/nchs/data/hus/2020-2021/VaxCh.pdf.

33 Hervé, Caroline, Béatrice Laupèze, Giuseppe Del Giudice, Arnaud M. Didierlaurent, and Fernanda Tavares Da Silva. "The How's and What's of Vaccine Reactogenicity." *NPJ Vaccines* 4, no. 1 (September 24, 2019). https://doi.org/10.1038/s41541-019-0132-6.

34 "Vaccine Schedule for Children 6 Years or Younger." Centers for Disease Control and Prevention, February 10, 2023. https://www.cdc.gov/vaccines/schedules/easy-to-read/child-easyread.html.

35 Mawson, Anthony R., and Ashley M. Croft. "Multiple Vaccinations and the Enigma of Vaccine Injury." *Vaccines* 8, no. 4 (2020): 676. https://doi.org/10.3390/vaccines8040676.

36 Fairbrother, Gerry, Elena Fuentes-Afflick, Lainie Friedman Ross, and Pauline A. Thomas. "Communicating with Parents About Immunization Safety: Messages for Pediatricians in the IOM Report 'The Childhood Immunization Schedule and Safety: Stakeholder Concerns, Scientific Evidence, and Future Studies.'" *Academic Pediatrics* 13, no. 5 (2013): 387–89. https://doi.org/10.1016/j.acap.2013.06.002.

37 Miller, Neil Z., and Gary S. Goldman. "Infant Mortality Rates Regressed Against Number of Vaccine Doses Routinely given: Is There a Biochemical or Synergistic Toxicity?" *Human And Experimental Toxicology* 30, no. 9 (2011): 1420–28. https://doi.org/10.1177/0960327111407644.

38 "Autism and Vaccines." Centers for Disease Control and Prevention, December 1, 2021. https://www.cdc.gov/vaccinesafety/concerns/autism.html.

39 Savage, Jessica, and Christina B. Johns. "Food Allergy: Epidemiology and Natural History." *Immunology and Allergy Clinics of North America,* February 2015. https://www.ncbi.nlm.nih.gov/pmc/articles/PMC4254585/.

40 Radhakrishnan, Dhenuka Kannan, Sharon D. Dell, Astrid Guttmann, Salimah Z. Shariff, Kuan Liu, and Teresa To. "Trends in the Age of Diagnosis of Childhood Asthma." *Journal of Allergy and Clinical Immunology* 134, no. 5 (2014). https://doi.org/10.1016/j.jaci.2014.05.012.

41 Kogan, Michael D., Catherine J. Vladutiu, Laura A. Schieve, Reem M. Ghandour, Stephen J. Blumberg, Benjamin Zablotsky, James M. Perrin, Karen A. Kuhlthau,

Robin L. Harwood, and Michael C. Lu. "The Prevalence of Parent-Reported Autism Spectrum Disorder among Us Children." *Pediatrics* 142, no. 6 (2018). https://doi.org/10.1542/peds.2017-4161.

42 Sharma, Samata R., Xenia Gonda, and Frank I. Tarazi. "Autism Spectrum Disorder: Classification, Diagnosis and Therapy." *Pharmacology & Therapeutics* 190 (2018): 91–104. https://doi.org/10.1016/j.pharmthera.2018.05.007.

43 "Autism and Vaccines." Centers for Disease Control and Prevention, December 1, 2021. https://www.cdc.gov/vaccinesafety/concerns/autism.html.

44 Ibid.

45 "Autism Prevalence Is Now 1 in 36, Signifying the 22% Increase in Prevalence Rates Reported by the CDC since 2021." The Autism Community in Action, April 20, 2023. https://tacanow.org/press-release/autism-prevalence-is-now-1-in-36/.

46 "Autism and Vaccines." Centers for Disease Control and Prevention, December 1, 2021. https://www.cdc.gov/vaccinesafety/concerns/autism.html.

47 "Autism Prevalence Is Now 1 in 36, Signifying the 22% Increase in Prevalence Rates Reported by the CDC since 2021." The Autism Community in Action, April 20, 2023. https://tacanow.org/press-release/autism-prevalence-is-now-1-in-36/.

48 Blaxill, Mark, Toby Rogers, and Cynthia Nevison. Autism Tsunami: The Impact of Rising Prevalence on the Societal Cost of Autism in the United States. *Science, Public Health Policy, and the Law.* 4 (December 2023): 227-256. https://www.publichealthpolicyjournal.com/_files/ugd/adf864_231644ca239249dc9ac579b5d332d872.pdf.

49 "Birth-18 Years Immunization Schedule, by Medical Condition." Centers for Disease Control and Prevention, November 16, 2023. https://www.cdc.gov/vaccines/schedules/hcp/imz/child-indications.html.

50 "Understanding Statistics: Risk." *BMJ* Best Practice. Accessed January 24, 2024. https://bestpractice.bmj.com/info/us/toolkit/learn-ebm/how-to-calculate-risk/#:

51 Niewiesk, Stefan. "Maternal Antibodies: Clinical Significance, Mechanism of Interference with Immune Responses, and Possible Vaccination Strategies." *Frontiers in Immunology* 5 (September 16, 2014). https://doi.org/10.3389/fimmu.2014.00446.

52 Ibid.

53 Njie-Jobe, Jainaba, Samuel Nyamweya, David J.C. Miles, Marianne van der Sande, Syed Zaman, Ebrima Touray, Safayet Hossin, et al. "Immunological Impact of an Additional Early Measles Vaccine in Gambian Children: Responses to a Boost at 3 Years." *Vaccine* 30, no. 15 (March 2012): 2543–50. https://doi.org/10.1016/j.vaccine.2012.01.083.

54 Niewiesk, Stefan. "Maternal Antibodies: Clinical Significance, Mechanism of Interference with Immune Responses, and Possible Vaccination Strategies." *Frontiers in Immunology* 5 (September 16, 2014). https://doi.org/10.3389/fimmu.2014.00446.

55 Haley Gans, Ross DeHovitz, Bagher Forghani, Judith Beeler, Yvonne Maldonado, and Ann M Arvin. "Measles and Mumps Vaccination as a Model to Investigate the Developing Immune System: Passive and Active Immunity During the First

Year of Life. *Vaccine* 21, no. 24 (July 28, 2003):3398-405. https://doi.org/10.1016/s0264-410x(03)00341-4.

56 "Polio Vaccine Trials Begin." This Day In History. Accessed January 24, 2024. https://www.history.com/this-day-in-history/polio-vaccine-trials-begin.

57 Merck & Co., Inc. Package Insert—VAXNEUVANCE. Food and Drug Administration (FDA), 2021. https://www.fda.gov/media/150819/download.

58 World Medical Association. "World Medical Association Declaration of Helsinki." *JAMA* 310, no. 20 (November 27, 2013): 2191. https://doi.org/10.1001/jama.2013.281053.

59 Alqahtani, Manaf, Saad I. Mallah, Nigel Stevenson, and Sally Doherty. "Vaccine Trials during a Pandemic: Potential Approaches to Ethical Dilemmas." *Trials* 22, no. 1 (2021). https://doi.org/10.1186/s13063-021-05597-8.

60 The Belmont Report: Ethical principles and guidelines for the Protection of Human Subjects of Research. 1978. US Department of Health and Human Services. https://www.hhs.gov/ohrp/regulations-and-policy/belmont-report/read-the-belmont-report/index.html.

61 "SIDS and Vaccines." Centers for Disease Control and Prevention, August 14, 2020. https://www.cdc.gov/vaccinesafety/concerns/sids.html.

62 Kogan, Michael D., Catherine J. Vladutiu, Laura A. Schieve, Reem M. Ghandour, Stephen J. Blumberg, Benjamin Zablotsky, James M. Perrin, et al. "The Prevalence of Parent-Reported Autism Spectrum Disorder among Us Children." *Pediatrics* 142, no. 6 (2018). https://doi.org/10.1542/peds.2017-4161.

63 Ibid.

64 Miller, Neil Z. "Vaccines and Sudden Infant Death: An Analysis of the VAERS Database 1990–2019 and Review of the Medical Literature." *Toxicology Reports* 8 (2021): 1324–35. https://doi.org/10.1016/j.toxrep.2021.06.020.

65 Moro, Pedro L., Silvia Perez-Vilar, Paige Lewis, Marthe Bryant-Genevier, Hajime Kamiya, and Maria Cano. "Safety Surveillance of Diphtheria and Tetanus Toxoids and Acellular Pertussis (Dtap) Vaccines." *Pediatrics* 142, no. 1 (July 1, 2018). https://doi.org/10.1542/peds.2017-4171.

66 Moon, Rachel Y., Robert A. Darnall, Lori Feldman-Winter, Michael H. Goodstein, and Fern R. Hauck. "SIDS and Other Sleep-Related Infant Deaths: Evidence Base for 2016 Updated Recommendations for a Safe Infant Sleeping Environment." *Pediatrics* 138, no. 5 (November 1, 2016). https://doi.org/10.1542/peds.2016-2940.

67 Moro, Pedro L., Jorge Arana, Maria Cano, Paige Lewis, and Tom T. Shimabukuro. "Deaths Reported to the Vaccine Adverse Event Reporting System, United States, 1997–2013." *Clinical Infectious Diseases* 61, no. 6 (May 28, 2015): 980–87. https://doi.org/10.1093/cid/civ423.

68 Eriksen, Eileen M., Jeffrey A. Perlman, Alvin Miller, S. Michael Marcy, Hang Lee, Constance Vadheim, Kenneth M. Zangwill, et al. "Lack of Association between Hepatitis B Birth Immunization and Neonatal Death." *Pediatric Infectious Disease Journal* 23, no. 7 (July 2004): 656–62. https://doi.org/10.1097/01.inf.0000130953.08946.d0.

69 Stratton, Kathleen, Donna A. Almario, Theresa M. Wizemann, and Marie C. McCormick. "Immunization Safety Review: Vaccinations and Sudden Unexpected Death in Infancy." Washington (DC): National Academies Press (US); 2003. PMID: 25057654., 2003. https://doi.org/ DOI: 10.17226/10649.

70 Silvers, Linda E., Susan S. Ellenberg, Robert P. Wise, Frederick E. Varricchio, Gina T. Mootrey, and Marcel E. Salive. "The Epidemiology of Fatalities Reported to the Vaccine Adverse Event Reporting System 1990–1997." *Pharmacoepidemiology and Drug Safety* 10, no. 4 (June 2001): 279–85. https://doi.org/10.1002/pds.619.

71 Griffin, Marie R., Wayne A. Ray, John R. Livengood, and William Schaffner. "Risk of Sudden Infant Death Syndrome after Immunization with the Diphtheria–Tetanus–Pertussis Vaccine." *New England Journal of Medicine* 319, no. 10 (September 8, 1988): 618–23. https://doi.org/10.1056/nejm198809083191006.

72 "SIDS and Vaccines." Centers for Disease Control and Prevention, August 14, 2020. https://www.cdc.gov/vaccinesafety/concerns/sids.html#rel/

73 Bethell, Christina D., Michael D. Kogan, Bonnie B. Strickland, Edward L. Schor, Julie Robertson, and Paul W. Newacheck. "A National and State Profile of Leading Health Problems and Health Care Quality for US Children: Key Insurance Disparities and across-State Variations." *Academic Pediatrics* 11, no. 3 (May 2011). https://doi.org/10.1016/j.acap.2010.08.011.

74 Hooker, Brian S., and Neil Z. Miller. "Analysis of Health Outcomes in Vaccinated and Unvaccinated Children: Developmental Delays, Asthma, Ear Infections and Gastrointestinal Disorders." *SAGE Open Medicine* 8 (January 2020). https://doi.org/10.1177/2050312120925344.

75 Ibid.

76 "Brain Architecture." Center on the Developing Child at Harvard University, August 20, 2019. https://developingchild.harvard.edu/science/key-concepts/brain-architecture/.

77 "A Common-Sense Approach to Childhood Vaccines Is Now Needed." World Council for Health, September 5, 2023. https://worldcouncilforhealth.org/news/statements/childhood-vaccines/.

Chapter 3

1 Arnold S. Relman and Marcia Angell. "America's Other Drug Problem: How the Drug Industry Distorts Medicine and Politics. *New Republic* 227, no. 25 (December 16, 2002): 27-41. PMID: 12561803. https://pubmed.ncbi.nlm.nih.gov/12561803/.

2 "How Vaccines are Developed and Approved for Use." Centers for Disease Control and Prevention. March 30, 2023. https://www.cdc.gov/vaccines/basics/test-approve.html.

3 Center for Drug Evaluation and Research. "New Drug Application (NDA)." Food and Drug Administration. January 21, 2022. https://www.fda.gov/drugs/types-applications/new-drug-application-nda.

4 Center for Biologics Evaluation And Research. "Biologics License Applications (BLA) Process (CBER)." U.S. Food And Drug Administration. January 27, 2021. https:

//www.fda.gov/vaccines-blood-biologics/development-approval-process-cber/biologics-license-applications-bla-process-cber.

5 ATrain Education. "4 Herd Immunity." Accessed January 20, 2024. https://www.atrainceu.com/content/4-herd-immunity.

Chapter 4

1 Washington Journal. "Influenza Vaccine." C-SPAN. October 11, 2004. Video, 49:22https://www.c-span.org/video/?183885-2/influenza-vaccine.

2 Appendix B for the Pink Book-Vaccine Excipient Summary. Accessed January 25, 2024. https://www.cdc.gov/vaccines/pubs/pinkbook/downloads/appendices/b/excipient-table-2.pdf.

3 "Interim Clinical Considerations for Use of COVID-19 Vaccines in the United States." Centers for Disease Control and Prevention. January 18, 2024. https://www.cdc.gov/vaccines/covid-19/clinical-considerations/interim-considerations-us.html#contraindications.

4 "Variation in the COVID-19 Infection–Fatality Ratio by Age, Time, and Geography during the Pre-Vaccine Era: A Systematic Analysis." *The Lancet* 399, no. 10334 (April 1, 2022): 1469–88. https://www.thelancet.com/journals/lancet/article/PIIS0140-6736(21)02867-1/fulltext.

5 Sorg, Anna-Lisa, Markus Hufnagel, Maren Doenhardt, Natalie Diffloth, Horst Schroten, R. Von Kries, Reinhard Berner, and Jakob Armann. "Risk of Hospitalization, Severe Disease, and Mortality Due to COVID-19 and PIMS-TS in Children with SARS-CoV-2 Infection in Germany." *MedRxiv (Cold Spring Harbor Laboratory)*, November 30, 2021. https://www.medrxiv.org/content/10.1101/2021.11.30.21267048v1.

6 American Academy of Pediatrics and the Children's Hospital Association. "COVID-19 and Age." August 5, 2021. https://downloads.aap.org/AAP/PDF/AAP%20and%20CHA%20-%20Children%20and%20COVID-19%20State%20Data%20Report%208.5%20FINAL.pdf.

7 FAIR Health, Inc. "Risk Factors for COVID-19 Mortality among Privately Insured Patients: A Claims Data Analysis." November 11, 2020. https://s3.amazonaws.com/media2.fairhealth.org/whitepaper/asset/Risk%20Factors%20for%20COVID-19%20Mortality%20among%20Privately%20Insured%20Patients%20-%20A%20Claims%20Data%20Analysis%20-%20A%20FAIR%20Health%20White%20Paper.pdf.

8 Smith, Caroline M., David Odd, Rachel Harwood, Joseph Ward, Mike Linney, Matthew Clark, Dougal Hargreaves, et al. "Deaths in Children and Young People in England after SARS-CoV-2 Infection during the First Pandemic Year." *Nature Medicine* 28, no. 1 (November 11, 2021): 185–92. https://www.nature.com/articles/s41591-021-01578-1.

9 "CDC COVID Data Tracker: Pediatric Seroprevalence." Centers for Disease Control and Prevention. December 11, 2022. https://covid.cdc.gov/covid-data-tracker/#pediatric-seroprevalence.

10 Karron, Ruth A., Maria Garcia Quesada, Elizabeth Schappell, Stephen D. Schmidt, Maria Deloria Knoll, Marissa K. Hetrich, Vic Veguilla, Nicole A. Doria-Rose, and Fatimah S. Dawood. "Binding and Neutralizing Antibody Responses to SARS-CoV-2 in Very Young Children Exceed Those in Adults." *JCI Insight* 7, no. 8 (April 22, 2022). https://insight.jci.org/articles/view/157963.

11 Altarawneh, Heba N., Hiam Chemaitelly, Houssein H. Ayoub, Mohammad Rubayet Hasan, Peter Coyle, Hadi M. Yassine, Hebah A. Al-Khatib, et al. "Protection of SARS-CoV-2 Natural Infection against Reinfection with the Omicron BA.4 or BA.5 Subvariants." *MedRxiv (Cold Spring Harbor Laboratory)*, July 12, 2022 https://www.medrxiv.org/content/10.1101/2022.07.11.22277448v1.

12 Stauffer, Elizabeth. "Johns Hopkins Doc Says Natural Immunity 27 Times More Effective than Vaccine." *The Western Journal*, November 2, 2021. https://www.westernjournal.com/johns-hopkins-doc-says-natural-immunity-27-times-effective-vaccine/.

13 Uusküla, Anneli, Heti Pisarev, Anna Tisler, Tatjana Meister, Kadri Suija, Kristi Huik, Aare Abroi, Ruth Kalda, Raivo Kolde, and Krista Fischer. "Risk of SARS-COV-2 Infection and Hospitalization in Individuals with Natural, Vaccine-Induced and Hybrid Immunity: A Retrospective Population-Based Cohort Study from Estonia." *Scientific Reports* 13, no. 1 (November 21, 2023). https://doi.org/10.1038/s41598-023-47043-6.

14 "Measles, Mumps, and Rubella (MMR) Vaccination." Centers for Disease Control and Prevention, January 26, 2021. https://www.cdc.gov/vaccines/vpd/mmr/public/index.html.

15 "Chickenpox Vaccination: What Everyone Should Know." Centers for Disease Control and Prevention, April 28, 2021. https://www.cdc.gov/vaccines/vpd/varicella/public/index.html.

16 Lin, Dan-Yu, Yu Gu, Yangjianchen Xu, Donglin Zeng, Bradford Wheeler, Hayley Young, Shadia Khan Sunny, and Zack Moore. "Effects of Vaccination and Previous Infection on Omicron Infections in Children." *New England Journal of Medicine* 387, no. 12 (September 22, 2022): 1141–43. https://doi.org/10.1056/nejmc2209371.

17 Shrestha, Nabin K., Patrick C. Burke, Amy S. Nowacki, James F. Simon, Amanda Hagen, and Steven M. Gordon. "Effectiveness of the Coronavirus Disease 2019 Bivalent Vaccine." *Open Forum Infectious Diseases* 10, no. 6 (April 19, 2023). https://doi.org/10.1093/ofid/ofad209.

18 Hansen, Christian Holm, Astrid Blicher Schelde, Ida Rask Moustsen-Helm, Hanne-Dorthe Emborg, Tyra Grove Krause, Kåre Mølbak, and Palle Valentiner-Branth. "Vaccine Effectiveness against SARS-COV-2 Infection with the Omicron or Delta Variants Following a Two-Dose or Booster BNT162b2 or mRNA-1273 Vaccination Series: A Danish Cohort Study." *MedRxiv*, December 21, 2021. https://doi.org/10.1101/2021.12.20.21267966.

19 "Risk Assessment Summary for SARS COV-2 Sublineage BA.2.86." Centers for Disease Control and Prevention, August 23, 2023. https://www.cdc.gov/respiratory-viruses/whats-new/covid-19-variant.html.

20 Puhach, Olha, Kenneth Adea, Nicolas Hulo, Pascale Sattonnet, Camille Genecand, Anne Iten, Frédérique Jacquérioz, et al. "Infectious Viral Load in Unvaccinated and Vaccinated Individuals Infected with Ancestral, Delta or Omicron Sars-COV-2." *Nature Medicine* 28, no. 7 (April 8, 2022): 1491–1500. https://doi.org/10.1038/s41591-022-01816-0.

21 Singanayagam, Anika, Seran Hakki, Jake Dunning, Kieran J. Madon, Michael A. Crone, Aleksandra Koycheva, Nieves Derqui-Fernandez, et al. "Community Transmission and Viral Load Kinetics of the SARS-COV-2 Delta (b.1.617.2) Variant in Vaccinated and Unvaccinated Individuals in the UK: A Prospective, Longitudinal, Cohort Study." *The Lancet Infectious Diseases* 22, no. 2 (February 2022): 183–95. https://doi.org/10.1016/s1473-3099(21)00648-4.

22 Haroun, Azmi, and Hilary Brueck. "CDC Director Says Data 'Suggests That Vaccinated People Do Not Carry the Virus.'" *Business Insider*, March 30, 2021. https://www.businessinsider.com/cdc-director-data-vaccinated-people-do-not-carry-covid-19-2021-3.

23 Choi, Joseph. "Fauci: Vaccinated People Become 'Dead Ends' for the Coronavirus." The Hill, May 16, 2021. https://thehill.com/homenews/sunday-talk-shows/553773-fauci-vaccinated-people-become-dead-ends-for-the-coronavirus/.

24 Kumar, Nikhilesh, Eran Bendavid, and Neeraj Sood. "Duration of SARS-COV-2 Culturable Virus Shedding in Children." *JAMA Pediatrics* 177, no. 12 (December 1, 2023): 1352. https://doi.org/10.1001/jamapediatrics.2023.4511.

25 Ibid.

26 Office of the Commissioner. "FDA Takes Key Action in Fight against COVID-19 by Issuing Emergency Use Authorization for First COVID-19 Vaccine." U.S. Food and Drug Administration, 2020. https://www.fda.gov/news-events/press-announcements/fda-takes-key-action-fight-against-covid-19-issuing-emergency-use-authorization-first-covid-19.

27 "Pfizer and BioNTech Receive U.S. FDA Approval for 2023-2024 COVID-19 Vaccine." Pfizer, September 11, 2023. https://www.pfizer.com/news/press-release/press-release-detail/pfizer-and-biontech-receive-us-fda-approval-2023-2024-covid

28 Bruce Yu, Yihua, Marc B. Taraban, and Katharine T. Briggs. "All Vials Are Not the Same: Potential Role of Vaccine Quality in Vaccine Adverse Reactions." *Vaccine* 39, no. 45 (October 2021): 6565–69. https://doi.org/10.1016/j.vaccine.2021.09.065.

29 Schmeling, Max, Vibeke Manniche, and Peter Riis Hansen. "Batch-dependent Safety of the BNT162B2 Mrna Covid-19 Vaccine." *European Journal of Clinical Investigation* 53, no. 8 (April 9, 2023). https://doi.org/10.1111/eci.13998.

30 Moderna US, Inc. *Package Insert—SPIKEVAX.* Food and Drug Administration (FDA), 2023. https://www.fda.gov/media/155675/download?attachment31

Munoz, F.M.; Sher, L.D.; Sabharwal, C.; Gurtman, A.; Xu, X.; Kitchin, N.; Lockhart, S.; Riesenberg, R.; Sexter, J.M.; Czajka, H.; et al. Evaluation of BNT162b2 COVID-19 Vaccine in Children Younger than 5 Years of Age. *N. Engl. J. Med.* 2023, *388*, 621–634. https://www.nejm.org/doi/full/10.1056/NEJMoa2211031.

32 Ibid.

33 FDA Briefing Document. "EUA amendment request for Pfizer-BioNTech COVID-19 Vaccine for use in children 6 months through 4 years of age." Vaccines and Related Biological Products Advisory Committee Meeting June 15, 2022. https://www.fda.gov/media/159195/download.

34 Pfizer-BioNTech COVID-19 Vaccine (2023-2024 Formula) authorized for individuals 6 months through 11 years of age. US Food and Drug Administration, Coronavirus-19, CBER-Regulated Biologics. December 11, 2023 https://www.fda.gov/vaccines-blood-biologics/coronavirus-covid-19-cber-regulated-biologics/pfizer-biontech-covid-19-vaccine.

35 Tirrell, Meg. "FDA Advisers Recommend That Covid-19 Boosters for Fall Should Drop Original Strain." CNN, June 15, 2023. https://www.cnn.com/2023/06/15/health/fda-advisers-covid-19-boosters/index.html.

36 Anderson, Steve. "CBR Plans for Monitoring COVID-19 Vaccine Safety and Effectiveness. VRBPAC Meeting, October 22, 2020. https://www.fda.gov/media/143557/download?fbclid=IwAR1SooRjTDuhBPqM4TiD3O7vYgX4eAp3CCqB7SzCk04CMve_OzgtMNPfNkc&utm_source=substack&utm_medium=email.

37 Jha, Ashish. "Press Briefing by White House COVID-19 Response Team and Public Health Officials." White House Press Briefing. June 23, 2022. https://www.whitehouse.gov/briefing-room/press-briefings/2022/06/23/press-briefing-by-white-house-covid-19-response-team-and-public-health-officials-86/.

38 Carnahan, Ashley. "CDC Could Add COVID Vaccine Requirement for Children to Immunization List with 'No Clinical Data': Dr. Makary." Fox News, October 19, 2022. https://www.foxnews.com/media/cdc-could-add-covid-vaccine-requirement-children-immunization-list-no-clinical-data-dr-makary.

39 Acevedo-Whitehouse, K., and R. Bruno. "Potential Health Risks of Mrna-Based Vaccine Therapy: A Hypothesis." *Medical Hypotheses* 171 (February 2023): 111015. https://doi.org/10.1016/j.mehy.2023.111015.

40 Polack, Fernando P., Stephen J. Thomas, Nicholas Kitchin, Judith Absalon, Alejandra Gurtman, Stephen Lockhart, John L. Perez, et al. "Safety and Efficacy of the BNT162B2 Mrna Covid-19 Vaccine." *New England Journal of Medicine* 383, no. 27 (December 31, 2020): 2603–15. https://doi.org/10.1056/nejmoa2034577.

41 FDA Briefing Document: Vaccines and Related Biological Products Advisory Committee Meeting, December 17, 2020. https://www.fda.gov/media/144434/download.

42 Brown, Ronald B. "Relative Risk Reduction: Misinformative Measure in Clinical Trials and COVID-19 Vaccine Efficacy." *Dialogues in Health* 1 (December 2022): 100074. https://doi.org/10.1016/j.dialog.2022.100074.

43 Ibid.

44 "V-Safe." Centers for Disease Control and Prevention, January 22, 2024. https://www.cdc.gov/vaccinesafety/ensuringsafety/monitoring/v-safe/index.html.

45 "CDC Won't Track COVID Transmission Levels Anymore in Major Shift." ABC News, May 5, 2023. https://abcnews.go.com/Health/cdc-changing-covid-19-surveillance-public-health-emergency/story?id=99088244.

46 Siri & Glimstad LLP. "CDC's Covid-19 Vaccine V-Safe Data Released Pursuant to Court Order." PR Newswire, October 4, 2022. https://www.prnewswire.com/news-releases/cdcs-covid-19-vaccine-v-safe-data-released-pursuant-to-court-order-301639584.html.

47 McKernan, Kevin, Yvonne Helbert, Liam T. Kane, and Stephen McLaughlin. 2023. "Sequencing of Bivalent Moderna and Pfizer Mrna Vaccines Reveals Nanogram to Microgram Quantities of Expression Vector Dsdna Per Dose." OSF Preprints. April 10. doi:10.31219/osf.io/b9t7m. https://osf.io/preprints/osf/b9t7m.

48 Speicher, David & Rose, Jessica & Gutschi, Luz & Wiseman, David & McKernan, Kevin. (2023). "DNA fragments detected in COVID-19 vaccines in Canada. DNA fragments detected in monovalent and bivalent." Preprint. https://www.researchgate.net/publication/374870815_Speicher_DJ_et_al_DNA_fragments_detected_in_COVID-19_vaccines_in_Canada_DNA_fragments_detected_in_monovalent_and_bivalent.

49 Horwood, Matthew. "Exclusive: Health Canada Confirms Undisclosed Presence of DNA Sequence in Pfizer Shot." *The Epoch Times*, November 1, 2023. https://www.theepochtimes.com/world/exclusive-health-canada-confirms-undisclosed-presence-of-dna-sequence-in-pfizer-shot-5513277.

50 Speicher, David J., Jessica Rose, L. Maria Gutschi, David M.. Wiseman, and Kevin McKernan. "DNA fragments detected in monovalent and bivalent Pfizer/BioNTech and Moderna modRNA Covid-19 vaccines from Ontario, Canada: Exploratory dose response relationship with serious adverse events." OSF Preprints. October 19, 2023. https://doi.org/10.31219/osf.io/mjc97.

51 Ibid.

52 Ibid.

53 McKernan, Kevin, Yvonne Helbert, Liam T. Kane, and Stephen McLaughlin. "Sequencing of bivalent Moderna and pfizer mrna vaccines reveals nanogram to microgram quantities of expression vector dsdna per dose." OSF Preprints. April 10, 2023. https://doi.org/10.31219/osf.io/b9t7m.

54 Block, Jennifer. "Covid-19: Researchers Face Wait for Patient Level Data from Pfizer and Moderna Vaccine Trials." *BMJ* (July 12, 2022). https://doi.org/10.1136/bmj.o1731.

55 Flowers, Chris, Erica Delph, and Ed Clark. "Report 86: Pfizer's Clinical Trial 'process 2' COVID Vaccine Recipients Suffered 2.4x the Adverse Events of Placebo Recipients; 'Process 2' Vials Were Contaminated with DNA Plasmids." DailyClout, October 26, 2023. https://dailyclout.io/pfizer-process-2-vaccine-had-2-4-times-adverse-events/.

56 "Florida State Surgeon General Calls for Halt in the Use of COVID-19 Mrna Vaccines." Florida Department of Health, Office of Communications. January 3, 2024. Accessed January 24, 2024. https://www.floridahealth.gov/newsroom/2024/01/20240103-halt-use-covid19-mrna-vaccines.pr.html.

57 "Guidance for Industry: Considerations for Plasmid DNA Vaccines for Infectious Disease Indications." U.S. Department of Health and Human Services, Food and Drug Administration, Center for Biologics Evaluation and Research. November 2007. https://www.fda.gov/media/73667/download?utm_source=floridahealth.go

v&utm_medium=referral&utm_campaign=PressRelease&utm_content=Florida%27s_Future_Budget&url_trace_7f2r5y6=Press_Release_Template_fry_2023_alt.docx.

58 Fujimori, Sachi. "Unlocking the Power of our Body's Protein Factory." June 2022. https://www.pfizer.com/news/behind-the-science/unlocking-power-our-bodys-protein-factory#:

59 "Florida State Surgeon General Calls for Halt in the Use of COVID-19 mRNA Vaccines." Florida Department of Health, Office of Communications. January 03, 2024. https://www.floridahealth.gov/newsroom/2024/01/20240103-halt-use-covid19-mrna-vaccines.pr.html.

60 Impelli, Matthew. "FDA Defends COVID Vaccine Against Smoking Gun Claims." Newsweek. November 01, 2023. https://www.newsweek.com/fda-defends-covid-vaccine-against-smoking-gun-claims-1840050.

61 Parry, Peter I., Astrid Lefringhausen, Conny Turni, Christopher J. Neil, Robyn Cosford, Nicholas J. Hudson, and Julian Gillespie. 2023. "'Spikeopathy': COVID-19 Spike Protein Is Pathogenic, from Both Virus and Vaccine mRNA." *Biomedicines* 11, no. 8: 2287. https://doi.org/10.3390/biomedicines11082287.

62 Ramachandra, Naik. "Summary Basis for Regulatory Action." May 18, 2021. https://www.fda.gov/media/151733/download.

63 "Myocarditis and Pericarditis after mRNA COVID-19 Vaccination." Centers for Disease Control and Prevention. Accessed January 24, 2024. https://www.cdc.gov/coronavirus/2019-ncov/vaccines/safety/myocarditis.html.

64 Tuvali, Ortal, Sagi Tshori, Estela Derazne, Rebecca Regina Hannuna, Arnon Afek, Dan Haberman, Gal Sella, and Jacob George. "The Incidence of Myocarditis and Pericarditis in Post Covid-19 Unvaccinated Patients—a Large Population-Based Study." *Journal of Clinical Medicine* 11, no. 8 (April 15, 2022): 2219. https://doi.org/10.3390/jcm11082219.

65 Mansanguan, Suyanee, Prakaykaew Charunwatthana, Watcharapong Piyaphanee, Wilanee Dechkhajorn, Akkapon Poolcharoen, and Chayasin Mansanguan. "Cardiovascular Manifestation of the BNT162B2 Mrna Covid-19 Vaccine in Adolescents." *Tropical Medicine and Infectious Disease* 7, no. 8 (August 19, 2022): 196. https://doi.org/10.3390/tropicalmed7080196.

66 Sharff, Katie A., David M. Dancoes, Jodi L. Longueil, Eric S. Johnson, and Paul F. Lewis. "Risk of Myopericarditis Following Covid-19 Mrna Vaccination in a Large Integrated Health System: A Comparison of Completeness and Timeliness of Two Methods." *Pharmacoepidemiology and Drug Safety* 31, no. 8 (April 16, 2022): 921–25. https://doi.org/10.1002/pds.5439.

67 Mansanguan, Suyanee, Prakaykaew Charunwatthana, Watcharapong Piyaphanee, Wilanee Dechkhajorn, Akkapon Poolcharoen, and Chayasin Mansanguan. "Cardiovascular Manifestation of the BNT162B2 Mrna Covid-19 Vaccine in Adolescents." *Tropical Medicine and Infectious Disease* 7, no. 8 (August 19, 2022): 196. https://doi.org/10.3390/tropicalmed7080196.

68 Hviid, Anders, Tuomo A Nieminen, Nicklas Pihlström, Nina Gunnes, Jesper Dahl, Øystein Karlstad, Hanne Løvdal Gulseth, Anders Sundström, Anders Husby,

Jørgen Vinsløv Hansen, Rickard Ljung, Petteri Hovi, "Booster vaccination with SARS-CoV-2 mRNA vaccines and myocarditis in adolescents and young adults: a Nordic cohort study." *European Heart Journal* 45, no. 7 (February 15, 2024): 1–9. https://doi.org/10.1093/eurheartj/ehae056.

69 Yu, Clement Kwong-man, Sabrina Tsao, Carol Wing-kei Ng, Gilbert T. Chua, Kwok-lap Chan, Julia Shi, Yumi Yuk-ting Chan, Patrick Ip, Mike Yat-wah Kwan, and Yiu-fai Cheung. "Cardiovascular Assessment up to One Year after COVID-19 Vaccine–Associated Myocarditis." Circulation 148, no. 5 (August 2023): 436–39. https://doi.org/10.1161/circulationaha.123.064772.

70 Ibid.

71 Mansanguan, Suyanee, Prakaykaew Charunwatthana, Watcharapong Piyaphanee, Wilanee Dechkhajorn, Akkapon Poolcharoen, and Chayasin Mansanguan. "Cardiovascular Manifestation of the BNT162B2 Mrna Covid-19 Vaccine in Adolescents." *Tropical Medicine and Infectious Disease* 7, no. 8 (August 19, 2022): 196. https://doi.org/10.3390/tropicalmed7080196.

72 Arola, Anita, Essi Pikkarainen, Jussi OT Sipilä, Jouni Pykäri, Päivi Rautava, and Ville Kytö. "Occurrence and Features of Childhood Myocarditis: A Nationwide Study in Finland." *Journal of the American Heart Association* 6, no. 11 (November 2017). https://doi.org/10.1161/jaha.116.005306.

73 Kang, Michael, Venu Chippa, and Jason An. "Viral Myocarditis." Treasure Island, FL: StatPearls Publishing, 2023. https://www.ncbi.nlm.nih.gov/books/NBK459259/.

74 Hulscher, Nicolas, Roger Hodkinson, William Makis, and Peter A. McCullough. "Autopsy Findings in Cases of Fatal Covid-19 Vaccine-induced Myocarditis." *ESC Heart Failure* (January 14, 2024). https://doi.org/10.1002/ehf2.14680.

75 Salsone, Maria, Carlo Signorelli, Alessandro Oldani, Valerio Fabio Alberti, Vincenza Castronovo, Salvatore Mazzitelli, Massimo Minerva, and Luigi Ferini-Strambi. "Neuro-COVAX: An Italian Population-Based Study of Neurological Complications after Covid-19 Vaccinations." *Vaccines* 11, no. 10 (October 21, 2023): 1621. https://doi.org/10.3390/vaccines11101621.

76 Ibid.

77 Garg, Ravindra Kumar, and Vimal Kumar Paliwal. "Spectrum of Neurological Complications Following COVID-19 Vaccination." *Neurological Sciences* 43, no. 1 (October 31, 2021): 3–40. https://doi.org/10.1007/s10072-021-05662-9.

78 Chatterjee, Aparajita, and Ambar Chakravarty. "Neurological Complications Following Covid-19 Vaccination." *Current Neurology and Neuroscience Reports* 23, no. 1 (November 29, 2022): 1–14. https://doi.org/10.1007/s11910-022-01247-x.

79 American Academy of Neurology. (2021) American Academy of Neurology Position Statement on COVID-19 Vaccination. https://www.aan.com/advocacy/covid-19-vaccination-position-statement.

80 "Covid-19 Vaccine for Children." American Academy of Pediatrics. Accessed January 24, 2024. https://www.aap.org/en/pages/2019-novel-coronavirus-covid-19-infections/covid-19-vaccine-for-children/.

81 Makis, William. "Children mRNA Injured—Encephalitis After Pfizer COVID-19 Mrna Vaccine—Potentially Deadly Brain Inflammation—33

Cases (Personality Changes, Seizures, Hallucinations)—3 Deaths, 4 Disabled." makismd.substack.com, November 24, 2023. https://makismd.substack.com/p/children-mrna-injured-encephalitis.

82 Erdogan, Mumin Alper, Orkun Gurbuz, Mehmet Fatih Bozkurt, and Oytun Erbas. "Prenatal Exposure to COVID-19 Mrna Vaccine BNT162B2 Induces Autism-like Behaviors in Male Neonatal Rats: Insights into Wnt and BDNF Signaling Perturbations." *Neurochemical Research*, January 10, 2024. https://doi.org/10.1007/s11064-023-04089-2.

83 Jaswa, Eleni G., Marcelle I. Cedars, Karla J. Lindquist, Somer L. Bishop, Young-Shin Kim, Amy Kaing, Mary Prahl, et al. "In Utero Exposure to Maternal COVID-19 Vaccination and Offspring Neurodevelopment at 12 and 18 Months." *JAMA Pediatrics*, January 22, 2024. https://doi.org/10.1001/jamapediatrics.2023.5743.

84 Ibid.

85 Lee, Katharine M., Eleanor J. Junkins, Chongliang Luo, Urooba A. Fatima, Maria L. Cox, and Kathryn B. Clancy. "Investigating Trends in Those Who Experience Menstrual Bleeding Changes after SARS-COV-2 Vaccination." *Science Advances* 8, no. 28 (July 15, 2022). https://doi.org/10.1126/sciadv.abm7201.

86 Thorp, James A., Claire Rogers, Michael P. Deskevich, Stewart Tankersley, Albert Benavides, A., Megan D. Redshaw, and Peter A. McCullough. "COVID-19 Vaccines: The Impact on Pregnancy Outcomes and Menstrual Function." *Journal of American Physicians and Surgeons*. 28, no. 1 (December 30, 2022). https://www.jpands.org/vol28no1/thorp.pdf.

87 Gat, Itai, Alon Kedem, Michal Dviri, Ana Umanski, Matan Levi, Ariel Hourvitz, and Micha Baum. "Covid-19 Vaccination BNT162B2 Temporarily Impairs Semen Concentration and Total Motile Count among Semen Donors." *Andrology* 10, no. 6 (June 27, 2022): 1016–22. https://doi.org/10.1111/andr.13209.

88 Renner, Vanessa. "Data Analyst Suggests COVID Jabs Linked to Steep Birth Rate Drop in Europe." LifeSite, September 15, 2022. https://www.lifesitenews.com/news/data-analyst-suggests-covid-jabs-linked-to-steep-birth-rate-drop-in-europe/.

89 Chudov, Igor. "Is Depopulation We Are Seeing, Planned or Incidental? December Births and Deaths Update." December 22, 2022. https://www.igor-chudov.com/p/is-depopulation-we-are-seeing-planned?utm_source=substack&utm_medium=email.

90 Bujard, Martin, and Gunnar Andersson. "Fertility Declines near the End of the COVID-19 Pandemic: Evidence of the 2022 Birth Declines in Germany and Sweden." *European Journal of Population* 40, no. 1 (January 22, 2024). https://doi.org/10.1007/s10680-023-09689-w.

91 Brown, Amanda. "Pfizer's Own Study Finds Nanoparticles in Covid Vaccines Enter Organs." *Western Standard*, May 11, 2022. https://www.westernstandard.news/business/pfizer-s-own-study-finds-nanoparticles-in-covid-vaccines-enter-organs/article_5b3955f6-d146-11ec-a272-cf3264db392b.html.

92 Noé, Andrés, Thanh D. Dang, Christine Axelrad, Emma Burrell, Susie Germano, Sonja Elia, David Burgner, Kirsten P. Perrett, Nigel Curtis, and Nicole L. Messina. "BNT162B2 COVID-19 Vaccination in Children Alters Cytokine Responses to

Heterologous Pathogens and Toll-like Receptor Agonists." *Frontiers in Immunology* 14 (August 25, 2023). https://doi.org/10.3389/fimmu.2023.1242380.

93 Guy, Rebecca, Katherine L. Henderson, Juliana Coelho, Helen Hughes, Emily L. Mason, Sarah M. Gerver, Alicia Demirjian, et al. "Increase in Invasive Group a Streptococcal Infection Notifications, England, 2022." *Eurosurveillance* 28, no. 1 (January 5, 2023). https://doi.org/10.2807/1560-7917.es.2023.28.1.2200942.

94 Adams, Helen. "'Unprecedented' Uptick in Invasive Group A Strep Infections." Medical University of South Carolina, May 16, 2023. https://web.musc.edu/about/news-center/2023/05/16/unprecedented-uptick-in-invasive-group-a-strep-infections.

95 Ibid.

96 Valk, Anika M., Jim B.D. Keijser, Koos P.J. van Dam, Eileen W. Stalman, Luuk Wieske, Maurice Steenhuis, Laura Y.L. Kummer, et al. "Suppressed igg4 Class Switching in Dupilumab and TNF Inhibitor-treated Patients After Repeated SARS-COV-2 mRNA Vaccination." *MedRxiv.* October 2, 2023. https://doi.org/10.1101/2023.09.29.23296354.

97 Crescioli, Silvia, Isabel Correa, Panagiotis Karagiannis, Anna M. Davies, Brian J. Sutton, Frank O. Nestle, and Sophia N. Karagiannis. "IgG4 Characteristics and Functions in Cancer Immunity." *Current Allergy and Asthma Reports* 16, no. 1 (January 2016). https://doi.org/10.1007/s11882-015-0580-7.

98 Zhang, Xia, Hui Lu, Linyi Peng, Jiaxin Zhou, Mu Wang, Jieqiong Li, Zheng Liu, et al. "The Role of PD-1/PD-LS in the Pathogenesis of Igg4-Related Disease." *Rheumatology* 61, no. 2 (April 30, 2021): 815–25. https://doi.org/10.1093/rheumatology/keab360.

99 Murata, Kazuhiro, Naoki Nakao, Naoki Ishiuchi, Takafumi Fukui, Narutaka Katsuya, Wataru Fukumoto, Hiroko Oka, et al. "Four Cases of Cytokine Storm after COVID-19 Vaccination: Case Report." *Frontiers in Immunology* 13 (August 15, 2022). https://doi.org/10.3389/fimmu.2022.967226.

100 Nune A, Durkowski V, Pillay SS, Barman B, Elwell H, Bora K, Bilgrami S, Mahmood S, Babajan N, Venkatachalam S, Ottewell L, Manzo C. "New-Onset Rheumatic Immune-Mediated Inflammatory Diseases Following SARS-CoV-2 Vaccinations until May 2023: A Systematic Review." *Vaccines* (Basel). 11(10):1571 (Oct 8, 2023) https://www.ncbi.nlm.nih.gov/pmc/articles/PMC10610967/.

101 Chen, Yue, Zhiwei Xu, Peng Wang, Xiao-Mei Li, Zong-Wen Shuai, Dong-Qing Ye, and Hai-Feng Pan. "New-onset Autoimmune Phenomena Post-covid-19 Vaccination." *Immunology* 165, no. 4 (January 7, 2022): 386–401. https://doi.org/10.1111/imm.13443.

102 Hinterseher, Julia, Michael Hertl, and Dario Didona. "Autoimmune Skin Disorders and SARS-COV-2 Vaccination – a Meta-analysis." *JDDG: Journal der Deutschen Dermatologischen Gesellschaft* 21, no. 8 (May 23, 2023): 853–61. https://doi.org/10.1111/ddg.15114.

103 Nune, Arvind, Victor Durkowski, S. Sujitha Pillay, Bhupen Barman, Helen Elwell, Kaustubh Bora, Syed Bilgrami, et al. "New-Onset Rheumatic Immune-Mediated Inflammatory Diseases Following SARS-COV-2 Vaccinations until May 2023: A

Systematic Review." *Vaccines* 11, no. 10 (October 8, 2023): 1571. https://doi.org/10.3390/vaccines11101571.

104 Kuek, Annabel, Brian L. Hazleman, and Andrew J. Östör. "Immune-Mediated Inflammatory Diseases (Imids) and Biologic Therapy: A Medical Revolution." *Postgraduate Medical Journal* 83, no. 978 (April 1, 2007): 251–60. https://doi.org/10.1136/pgmj.2006.052688.

105 Lin, Dan-Yu, Yu Gu, Yangjianchen Xu, Donglin Zeng, Bradford Wheeler, Hayley Young, Shadia Khan Sunny, and Zack Moore. "Effects of Vaccination and Previous Infection on Omicron Infections in Children." *New England Journal of Medicine* 387, no. 12 (September 22, 2022): 1141–43. https://doi.org/10.1056/nejmc2209371.

106 Shrestha, Nabin K., Patrick C. Burke, Amy S. Nowacki, James F. Simon, Amanda Hagen, and Steven M. Gordon. "Effectiveness of the Coronavirus Disease 2019 Bivalent Vaccine." *Open Forum Infectious Diseases* 10, no. 6 (April 19, 2023). https://doi.org/10.1093/ofid/ofad209.

107 "Risk Assessment Summary for SARS CoV-2 Sublineage BA.2.86." Centers for Disease Control and Prevention, August 23, 2023. https://www.cdc.gov/respiratory-viruses/whats-new/covid-19-variant.html.

108 Puhach, Olha, Kenneth Adea, Nicolas Hulo, Pasacale Sattonnet, Camille Genecand, Anne Iten, Frederique Jacquerioz, et al. "Infectious viral load in unvaccinated and vaccinated individuals infected with ancestral, Delta or Omicron SARS-CoV-2." *Nature Medicine* 28, 1491–1500 (2022). https://doi.org/10.1038/s41591-022-01816-0.

Chapter 5

1 "Hepatitis B—Faqs, Statistics, Data, & Guidelines." Centers for Disease Control and Prevention, March 9, 2023. https://www.cdc.gov/hepatitis/hbv/index.htm.

2 "Hepatitis B Vaccination of Infants—Adolescents." Centers for Disease Control and Prevention, November 8, 2019. https://www.cdc.gov/hepatitis/hbv/vaccchildren.htm.

3 "Frequently Asked Questions for Health Professionals." Centers for Disease Control and Prevention, March 30, 2022. https://www.cdc.gov/hepatitis/hbv/hbvfaq.htm#D4.

4 Ibid.

5 Appendix B for the Pink Book-Vaccine Excipient Summary. Accessed January 25, 2024. https://www.cdc.gov/vaccines/pubs/pinkbook/downloads/appendices/b/excipient-table-2.pdf.

6 Ibid.

7 "ACIP Contraindications Guidelines for Immunization." Centers for Disease Control and Prevention, August 1, 2023. https://www.cdc.gov/vaccines/hcp/acip-recs/general-recs/contraindications.html.

8 "Screening and Testing Recommendations for Chronic Hepatitis B Virus Infection (HBV)| CDC." Centers for Disease Control and Prevention, March 28, 2022. https://www.cdc.gov/hepatitis/hbv/testingchronic.htm.

9 "Recommendations of the Immunization Practices Advisory Committee Prevention of Perinatal Transmission of Hepatitis B Virus: Prenatal Screening of All Pregnant Women for Hepatitis B Surface Antigen." Centers for Disease Control and Prevention, June 10, 1988. https://www.cdc.gov/mmwr/preview/mmwrhtml/00000036.htm#:.

10 Merck & Co., Inc. Package Insert: RECOMBIVAX HB. Food and Drug Administration (FDA), 2018. https://www.fda.gov/media/74274/download?attachment.

11 GlaxoSmithKline Biologicals. Package Insert: ENGERIX-B. Food and Drug Administration (FDA), 202X. https://www.fda.gov/media/119403/download?attachment.

12 Merck & Co., Inc. Package Insert: RECOMBIVAX HB. Food and Drug Administration (FDA), 2018. https://www.fda.gov/media/74274/download?attachment.

13 GlaxoSmithKline Biologicals. *Package Insert: ENGERIX-B.* 202X. https://www.fda.gov/media/119403/download?attachment.

14 Merck & Co., Inc. Package Insert: RECOMBIVAX HB. Food and Drug Administration (FDA), 2018. https://www.fda.gov/media/74274/download?attachment.

15 GlaxoSmithKline Biologicals. *Package Insert: ENGERIX-B.* Food and Drug Administration (FDA), 202X. https://www.fda.gov/media/119403/download?attachment.

16 "Prevention of Hepatitis B Virus Infection in the United States: Recommendations of the Advisory Committee on Immunization Practices." Centers for Disease Control and Prevention, May 22, 2018. https://www.cdc.gov/mmwr/volumes/67/rr/rr6701a1.htm.

17 Ibid.

18 GlaxoSmithKline Biologicals. *Package Insert: ENGERIX-B.* Food and Drug Administration (FDA), 202X. https://www.fda.gov/media/119403/download?attachment.

19 Ibid.

20 Lazarus, Ross. "Electronic Support for Public Health—Vaccine Adverse Event Reporting System (ESP:Vaers)." Digital Healthcare Research. Accessed January 24, 2024. https://digital.ahrq.gov/ahrq-funded-projects/electronic-support-public-health-vaccine-adverse-event-reporting-system.

21 GlaxoSmithKline Biologicals. *Package Insert: ENGERIX-B.* Food and Drug Administration (FDA), 202X. https://www.fda.gov/media/119403/download?attachment.

22 "Recommendations of the Immunization Practices Advisory Committee Prevention of Perinatal Transmission of Hepatitis B Virus: Prenatal Screening of All Pregnant Women for Hepatitis B Surface Antigen." Centers for Disease Control and Prevention, June 10, 1988. https://www.cdc.gov/mmwr/preview/mmwrhtml/00000036.htm#:

23 "Hepatitis B—Faqs, Statistics, Data, & Guidelines." Centers for Disease Control and Prevention, March 9, 2023. https://www.cdc.gov/hepatitis/hbv/index.htm.

24 Verstraeten, Thomas M., R. Davies, D. Gu, and F. DeStefano. "Increased Risk of Developmental Neurologic Impairment After High Exposure to Thimerosal-containing Vaccine in First Month of Life." https://vaccine-safety.s3.amazonaws.com/CDC_FOIA_Response_UnpublishedStudy.pdf.

Chapter 6

1 "RSV in Infants and Young Children." Centers for Disease Control and Prevention, January 18, 2024. https://www.cdc.gov/rsv/high-risk/infants-young-children.html.

2 Radhakrishnan, Rohini. "What Is the Mortality Rate of RSV in Babies?" MedicineNet, July 19, 2021. https://www.medicinenet.com/what_is_the_mortality_rate_of_rsv_in_babies/article.htm.

3 AstraZeneca. *Package Insert: BEYFORTUS*. Food and Drug Administration (FDA), July 2023. https://www.accessdata.fda.gov/drugsatfda_docs/label/2023/761328s000lbl.pdf.

4 "Symptoms and Care of RSV (Respiratory Syncytial Virus)." Centers for Disease Control and Prevention, September 6, 2023. https://www.cdc.gov/rsv/about/symptoms.html#:

5 Hansen, Chelsea L., Sandra S. Chaves, Clarisse Demont, and Cécile Viboud. "Mortality Associated with Influenza and Respiratory Syncytial Virus in the US, 1999-2018." *JAMA Network Open* 5, no. 2 (February 28, 2022). https://doi.org/10.1001/jamanetworkopen.2022.0527.

6 "RSV in Infants and Young Children." Centers for Disease Control and Prevention, January 18, 2024. https://www.cdc.gov/rsv/high-risk/infants-young-children.html.

7 Rogers, Lindsay Smith. "The Latest in RSV Protection for Kids: An Antibody Treatment Called Beyfortus." Johns Hopkins Bloomberg School of Public Health, July 27, 2023. https://publichealth.jhu.edu/2023/beyfortus-provides-rsv-protection-for-kids

8 "Monoclonal Antibodies: Definition & How Treatment Works." Cleveland Clinic, November 16, 2021. https://my.clevelandclinic.org/health/treatments/22246-monoclonal-antibodies.

9 Hammitt, Laura L., Ron Dagan, Yuan Yuan, Manuel Baca Cots, Miroslava Bosheva, Shabir A. Madhi, William J. Muller, et al. "Nirsevimab for Prevention of RSV in Healthy Late-Preterm and Term Infants." *New England Journal of Medicine* 386, no. 9 (March 3, 2022): 837–46. https://doi.org/10.1056/nejmoa2110275.

10 Ibid.

11 Astra Zeneca. *Package Insert: BEYFORTUS*. July 2023. https://products.sanofi.us/beyfortus/beyfortus.pdf.

12 Hammitt, Laura L., Ron Dagan, Yuan Yuan, Manuel Baca Cots, Miroslava Bosheva, Shabir A. Madhi, William J. Muller, et al. "Nirsevimab for Prevention of RSV in Healthy Late-Preterm and Term Infants." *New England Journal of Medicine* 386, no. 9 (March 3, 2022): 837–46. https://doi.org/10.1056/nejmoa2110275.

13 Keizer, Ron J., Alwin D.R. Huitema, Jan H.M. Schellens, and Jos H. Beijnen. "Clinical Pharmacokinetics of Therapeutic Monoclonal Antibodies." *Clinical Pharmacokinetics* 49, no. 8 (August 2010): 493–507. https://doi.org/10.2165/11531280-000000000-00000.

Chapter 7

1 Ruf, Bernhard R., and Markus Knuf. "The Burden of Seasonal and Pandemic Influenza in Infants and Children." *European Journal of Pediatrics* 173, no. 3 (May 10, 2013): 265–76. https://doi.org/10.1007/s00431-013-2023-6.

2 Boddington, Nicki L., Isabelle Pearson, Heather Whitaker, Punam Mangtani, and Richard G. Pebody. "Effectiveness of Influenza Vaccination in Preventing Hospitalization Due to Influenza in Children: A Systematic Review and Meta-Analysis." *Clinical Infectious Diseases* 73, no. 9 (March 27, 2021): 1722–32. https://doi.org/10.1093/cid/ciab270.

3 "Seasonal Influenza Vaccine Dosage & Administration." Centers for Disease Control and Prevention, November 16, 2020. https://www.cdc.gov/flu/about/qa/vaxadmin.htm.

4 "Different Types of Flu Vaccines." Centers for Disease Control and Prevention, August 31, 2022. https://www.cdc.gov/flu/prevent/different-flu-vaccines.htm.

5 "Cell-Based Flu Vaccines." Centers for Disease Control and Prevention, August 25, 2023. https://www.cdc.gov/flu/prevent/cell-based.htm.

6 "Vaccine Excipient Summary." Centers for Disease Control and Prevention, November 1, 2021. https://www.cdc.gov/vaccines/pubs/pinkbook/downloads/appendices/b/excipient-table-2.pdf.

7 "Summary of Recommendations." Centers for Disease Control and Prevention, August 23, 2023. https://www.cdc.gov/flu/pdf/professionals/acip/acip-2023-24-Summary-Flu-Vaccine-Recommendations.pdf.

8 "Flu Symptoms & Complications." Centers for Disease Control and Prevention, October 3, 2022. https://www.cdc.gov/flu/symptoms/symptoms.htm.

9 "Flu & People with Asthma." Centers for Disease Control and Prevention, September 6, 2022. https://www.cdc.gov/flu/highrisk/asthma.htm.

10 "Flu & Children with Neurologic Conditions." Centers for Disease Control and Prevention, November 30, 2022. https://www.cdc.gov/flu/highrisk/neurologic-pediatric.htm.

11 "Flu & Children at Higher Risk." Centers for Disease Control and Prevention, September 14, 2022. https://www.cdc.gov/flu/highrisk/children-high-risk.htm.

12 "Pediatric Flu Deaths during 2019-2020 Reach New High." Centers for Disease Control and Prevention, June 4, 2021. https://www.cdc.gov/flu/spotlights/2020-2021/pediatric-flu-deaths-reach-new-high.htm.

13 Ibid.

14 Sanofi Pasteur, Inc. *Package Insert: FLUZONE QUADRIVALENT.* Food and Drug Administration (FDA), July 2022. https://www.fda.gov/media/119856/download.

15 Ibid.

16 Ibid.

17 Carrat, F., A. Lavenu, S. Cauchemez, and S. Deleger. "Repeated Influenza Vaccination of Healthy Children and Adults: Borrow Now, Pay Later?" Epidemiology and Infection 134, no. 1 (November 21, 2005): 63–70. https://doi.org/10.1017/S0950268805005479.

18 Jefferson, Tom, Alessandro Rivetti, Carlo Di Pietrantonj, and Vittorio Demicheli. "Vaccines for Preventing Influenza in Healthy Children." *Cochrane Database of Systematic Reviews* 2018, no. 2 (February 1, 2018). https://doi.org/10.1002/14651858.cd004879.pub5.

19 Joshi, Avni Y., Vivek N. Iyer, Martha F. Hartz, Ashok M. Patel, and James T. Li. "Effectiveness of Trivalent Inactivated Influenza Vaccine in Influenza-Related Hospitalization in Children: A Case-Control Study." *Allergy and Asthma Proceedings* 33, no. 2 (March 1, 2012): 23–27. https://doi.org/10.2500/aap.2012.33.3513.

20 Cowling, Benjamin J., Vicky J. Fang, Hiroshi Nishiura, Kwok-Hung Chan, Sophia Ng, Dennis K. Ip, Susan S. Chiu, Gabriel M. Leung, and J. S. Peiris. "Increased Risk of Noninfluenza Respiratory Virus Infections Associated with Receipt of Inactivated Influenza Vaccine." *Clinical Infectious Diseases* 54, no. 12 (March 15, 2012): 1778–83. https://doi.org/10.1093/cid/cis307.

21 Doshi, Peter. "Influenza Vaccines." *JAMA Internal Medicine* 173, no. 11 (June 10, 2013): 1014. https://doi.org/10.1001/jamainternmed.2013.490.

22 https://www.midwesterndoctor.com/p/why-the-covid-vaccines-were-never.

23 Doshi, P. "Influenza: Marketing Vaccine by Marketing Disease." *BMJ* 346, no. 16 1 (May 16, 2013). https://doi.org/10.1136/bmj.f3037.

24 Jefferson, Tom, Alessandro Rivetti, Carlo Di Pietrantonj, Vittorio Demicheli, and Eliana Ferroni. "Vaccines for Preventing Influenza in Healthy Children." *Cochrane Database of Systematic Reviews* 8 (August 15, 2012). https://doi.org/10.1002/14651858.cd004879.pub4.

25 Jefferson, Tom, Alessandro Rivetti, Carlo Di Pietrantonj, and Vittorio Demicheli. "Vaccines for Preventing Influenza in Healthy Children." *Cochrane Database of Systematic Reviews* 2018, 2 (February 1, 2018). https://doi.org/10.1002/14651858.cd004879.pub5.

Chapter 8

1 Skibinski, David A.G., Barbara C. Baudner, Manmohan Singh, and Derek T. O'Hagan. "Combination Vaccines." *Journal of Global Infectious Diseases* 3, no. 1 (2011): 63. https://doi.org/10.4103/0974-777x.77298.

2 "Diphtheria, Tetanus, and Whooping Cough Vaccination: What You Should Know." Centers for Disease Control and Prevention, September 6, 2022. https://www.cdc.gov/vaccines/vpd/dtap-tdap-td/public/index.html.

3 "About Diphtheria, Tetanus, and Pertussis Vaccination." Centers for Disease Control and Prevention, September 6, 2022. https://www.cdc.gov/vaccines/vpd/dtap-tdap-td/hcp/about-vaccine.html.

4 "Vaccine Excipient Summary." Centers for Disease Control and Prevention, November 1, 2021. https://www.cdc.gov/vacines/pubs/pinkbook/downloads/appendices/b/excipient-table-2.pdf.

5 Ibid.

6 GlaxoSmithKline Biologicals. *Package Insert: INFARIX.* Food and Drug Administration (FDA), 2023. https://www.fda.gov/media/75157/download.

7 Sanofi Pasteur Limited. *Package Insert: DAPTAC.* Food and Drug Administration (FDA), 202X. https://www.fda.gov/media/74035/download.

8 "Safety Information for Diphtheria, Tetanus, and Pertussis Vaccines." Centers for Disease Control and Prevention, June 14, 2023. https://www.cdc.gov/vaccine safety/vaccines/dtap-tdap-vaccine.html#:

9 Moro, Pedro L., Silvia Perez-Vilar, Paige Lewis, Marthe Bryant-Genevier, Hajime Kamiya, and Maria Cano. "Safety Surveillance of Diphtheria and Tetanus Toxoids and Acellular Pertussis (Dtap) Vaccines." *Pediatrics* 142, no. 1 (July 1, 2018). https://doi.org/10.1542/peds.2017-4171.

10 Ibid.

11 Fraiman, Joseph, Juan Erviti, Mark Jones, Sander Greenland, Patrick Whelan, Robert M. Kaplan, and Peter Doshi. "Serious Adverse Events of Special Interest Following Mrna COVID-19 Vaccination in Randomized Trials in Adults." *Vaccine* 40, no. 40 (September 2022): 5798–5805. https://doi.org/10.1016/j .vaccine.2022.08.036.

12 Lazarus, Ross. "Electronic Support for Public Health—Vaccine Adverse Event Reporting System (ESP:Vaers)." Digital Healthcare Research. Accessed January 24, 2024. https://digital.ahrq.gov/ahrq-funded-projects/electronic-support-public -health-vaccine-adverse-event-reporting-system.

13 Moro, Pedro L., Silvia Perez-Vilar, Paige Lewis, Marthe Bryant-Genevier, Hajime Kamiya, and Maria Cano. "Safety Surveillance of Diphtheria and Tetanus Toxoids and Acellular Pertussis (Dtap) Vaccines." *Pediatrics* 142, no. 1 (July 1, 2018). https://doi.org/10.1542/peds.2017-4171.

14 Mercer, L., S. Creighton, J. J. Holden, and M. E. Lewis. "Parental Perspectives on the Causes of an Autism Spectrum Disorder in Their Children." Journal of Genetic Counseling 15, no. 1 (February 2006): 41–50. https://onlinelibrary.wiley. com/doi/10.1007/s10897-005-9002-7.

15 Geier, David A., and Mark R. Geier. "Neurodevelopmental Disorders Following Thimerosal-Containing Childhood Immunizations: A Follow-up Analysis." *International Journal of Toxicology* 23, no. 6 (November 2004): 369–76. https://doi .org/10.1080/10915810490902038.

16 Stratton, Kathleen R. *Adverse effects of vaccines: Evidence and causality.* Washington, D.C.: National Academies Press, 2012.

17 "About Diphtheria, Tetanus, and Pertussis Vaccination." Centers for Disease Control and Prevention, September 6, 2022. https://www.cdc.gov/vaccines/vpd /dtap-tdap-td/hcp/about-vaccine.html.

18 Tetanus.pdf. Accessed January 26, 2024. https://www.cdc.gov/vaccines/pubs /pinkbook/downloads/tetanus.pdf.

19 "About Diphtheria, Tetanus, and Pertussis Vaccination." Centers for Disease Control and Prevention, September 6, 2022. https://www.cdc.gov/vaccines/vpd/dtap-tdap -td/hcp/about-vaccine.html.

20 "Tetanus: For Clinicians." Centers for Disease Control and Prevention, August 29, 2022https://www.cdc.gov/tetanus/clinicians.html.

21 O'Brien, Judith A., and J. Jaime Caro. "Hospitalization for Pertussis: Profiles and Case Costs by Age." *BMC Infectious Diseases* 5, no. 1 (July 11, 2005). https://doi.org/10.1186/1471-2334-5-57.

22 "About Diphtheria, Tetanus, and Pertussis Vaccination." Centers for Disease Control and Prevention, September 6, 2022. https://www.cdc.gov/vaccines/vpd/dtap-tdap-td/hcp/about-vaccine.html.

23 "Pertussis Vaccination: Use of Acellular Pertussis Vaccines Among Infants and Young Children. Recommendations of the Advisory Committee on Immunization Practices (ACIP). (1997). *Recommendations and reports: Morbidity and Mortality Weekly Report* 46 (RR-7), 1–25. https://pubmed.ncbi.nlm.nih.gov/9091780/.

24 Misegades, Lara K., Kathleen Winter, Kathleen Harriman, John Talarico, Nancy E. Messonnier, Thomas A. Clark, and Stacey W. Martin. "Association of Childhood Pertussis with Receipt of 5 Doses of Pertussis Vaccine by Time since Last Vaccine Dose, California, 2010." *JAMA* 308, no. 20 (November 28, 2012): 2126. https://doi.org/10.1001/jama.2012.14939.

25 Zerbo, Ousseny, Joan Bartlett, Kristin Goddard, Bruce Fireman, Edwin Lewis, and Nicola P. Klein. "Acellular Pertussis Vaccine Effectiveness over Time." *Pediatrics* 144, no. 1 (June 10, 2019). https://doi.org/10.1542/peds.2018-3466.

26 Ibid.

27 GlaxoSmithKline Biologicals. *Package Insert: BOOSTRIX*. Food and Drug Administration (FDA), 2023. https://www.fda.gov/media/124002/download.

28 Decker, Michael D., and Kathryn M. Edwards. "Pertussis (Whooping Cough)." *Journal of Infectious Diseases* 224, no. Supplement_4 (September 30, 2021). https://doi.org/10.1093/infdis/jiaa469.

29 Liko, Juventila, Steve G. Robison, and Paul R. Cieslak. "Priming with Whole-Cell versus Acellular Pertussis Vaccine." *New England Journal of Medicine* 368, no. 6 (February 7, 2013): 581–82. https://doi.org/10.1056/nejmc1212006.

30 Witt, Maxwell A., Larry Arias, Paul H. Katz, Elizabeth T. Truong, and David J. Witt. "Reduced Risk of Pertussis among Persons Ever Vaccinated with Whole Cell Pertussis Vaccine Compared to Recipients of Acellular Pertussis Vaccines in a Large US Cohort." *Clinical Infectious Diseases* 56, no. 9 (March 13, 2013): 1248–54. https://doi.org/10.1093/cid/cit046.

31 Warfel, Jason M., Lindsey I. Zimmerman, and Tod J. Merkel. "Acellular Pertussis Vaccines Protect against Disease but Fail to Prevent Infection and Transmission in a Nonhuman Primate Model." *Proceedings of the National Academy of Sciences* 111, no. 2 (November 25, 2013): 787–92. https://doi.org/10.1073/pnas.1314688110.

32 Ibid.

33 Deen, J. L., C. M. Mink, J. D. Cherry, P. D. Christenson, E. F. Pineda, K. Lewis, D. A. Blumberg, and L. A. Ross. "Household Contact Study of Bordetella Pertussis Infections." *Clinical Infectious Diseases* 21, no. 5 (November 1, 1995): 1211–19. https://doi.org/10.1093/clinids/21.5.1211.

34 Warfel, Jason M., Lindsey I. Zimmerman, and Tod J. Merkel. "Acellular Pertussis Vaccines Protect against Disease but Fail to Prevent Infection and Transmission in

a Nonhuman Primate Model." *Proceedings of the National Academy of Sciences* 111, no. 2 (November 25, 2013): 787–92. https://doi.org/10.1073/pnas.1314688110.

35 Ibid.

36 Sanofi Pasteur Limited. *Package Insert: DAPTACEL.* Food and Drug Administration (FDA), 202X. https://www.fda.gov/media/74035/download.

37 GlaxoSmithKline Biologicals. *Package Insert: INFANRIX.* Food and Drug Administration (FDA), 2023. https://www.fda.gov/media/75157/download.

38 Misegades, Lara K., Kathleen Winter, Kathleen Harriman, John Talarico, Nancy E. Messonnier, Thomas A. Clark, and Stacey W. Martin. "Association of Childhood Pertussis with Receipt of 5 Doses of Pertussis Vaccine by Time since Last Vaccine Dose, California, 2010." *JAMA* 308, no. 20 (November 28, 2012): 2126. https://doi.org/10.1001/jama.2012.14939.

39 Zerbo, Ousseny, Joan Bartlett, Kristin Goddard, Bruce Fireman, Edwin Lewis, and Nicola P. Klein. "Acellular Pertussis Vaccine Effectiveness over Time." *Pediatrics* 144, no. 1 (June 10, 2019). https://doi.org/10.1542/peds.2018-3466.

40 Klein, Nicola P., Joan Bartlett, Bruce Fireman, Laurie Aukes, Philip O. Buck, Girishanthy Krishnarajah, and Roger Baxter. "Waning Protection Following 5 Doses of a 3-Component Diphtheria, Tetanus, and Acellular Pertussis Vaccine." *Vaccine* 35, no. 26 (June 2017): 3395–3400. https://doi.org/10.1016/j.vaccine.2017.05.008.

41 Klein, Nicola P., Joan Bartlett, Ali Rowhani-Rahbar, Bruce Fireman, and Roger Baxter. "Waning Protection after Fifth Dose of Acellular Pertussis Vaccine in Children." *New England Journal of Medicine* 367, no. 11 (September 13, 2012): 1012–19. https://doi.org/10.1056/nejmoa1200850.

42 Cherry, James D. "The 112-Year Odyssey of Pertussis and Pertussis Vaccines—Mistakes Made and Implications for the Future." *Journal of the Pediatric Infectious Diseases Society* 8, no. 4 (February 22, 2019): 334–41. https://doi.org/10.1093/jpids/piz005.

43 Ibid.

44 "Pregnancy & Vaccines." Centers for Disease Control and Prevention, September 29, 2023. https://www.cdc.gov/vaccines/parents/by-age/pregnancy.html.

Chapter 9

1 "Measles (Rubeola)." Centers for Disease Control and Prevention, November 5, 2020. https://www.cdc.gov/measles/index.html.

2 "Mumps." Centers for Disease Control and Prevention, March 8, 2021. https://www.cdc.gov/mumps/index.html.

3 "Rubella (German Measles)." Centers for Disease Control and Prevention, December 31, 2020. https://www.cdc.gov/rubella/index.html.

4 "Measles, Mumps, and Rubella (MMR) Vaccination." Centers for Disease Control and Prevention, January 26, 2021. https://www.cdc.gov/vaccines/vpd/mmr/public/index.html.

5 "U.S. Vaccine Names." Centers for Disease Control and Prevention, March 26, 2019. https://www.cdc.gov/vaccines/terms/usvaccines.html.

6 "Measles, Mumps, and Rubella (MMR) Vaccination." Centers for Disease Control and Prevention, January 26, 2021. https://www.cdc.gov/vaccines/vpd/mmr/public/index.html.

7 "Vaccine Excipient Summary." Centers for Disease Control and Prevention, November 1, 2021. https://www.cdc.gov/vaccines/pubs/pinkbook/downloads/appendices/b/excipient-table-2.pdf.

8 Ibid.

9 "ACIP Contraindications Guidelines for Immunization." Centers for Disease Control and Prevention, August 1, 2023. https://www.cdc.gov/vaccines/hcp/acip-recs/general-recs/contraindications.html.

10 Orenstein, Walter A., Alan R. Hinman, and Mark J. Panpania, eds. "Evolution of Measles Elimination Strategies in the United States." *Journal of Infectious Diseases* 189, no. Supplement_1 (May 1, 2004). https://doi.org/10.1086/377694.

11 "Rate of Cases and Deaths from Measles in the United States." Our World in Data. Accessed March 29, 2024. https://ourworldindata.org/grapher/measles-cases-and-death-rate.

12 "Measles Signs and Symptoms." Centers for Disease Control and Prevention, November 5, 2020. https://www.cdc.gov/measles/symptoms/signs-symptoms.html

13 "Measles Complications." Centers for Disease Control and Prevention, November 5, 2020. https://www.cdc.gov/measles/symptoms/complications.html.

14 "Pinkbook: Rubella." Centers for Disease Control and Prevention, August 18, 2021. https://www.cdc.gov/vaccines/pubs/pinkbook/rubella.html#rubella-vaccine.

15 Merck Sharp & Dohme LLC. *Package Insert: M-M-R II.* Food and Drug Administration (FDA), August, 2023. https://www.fda.gov/media/75191/download.

16 "Autism and Vaccines." Centers for Disease Control and Prevention, December 1, 2021. https://www.cdc.gov/vaccinesafety/concerns/autism.html.

17 "About Measles Vaccination." Centers for Disease Control and Prevention, January 26, 2021. https://www.cdc.gov/vaccines/vpd/measles/index.html

18 Merck Sharp & Dohme LLC. *Package Insert*: M-M-R II. Food and Drug Administration (FDA), August, 2023https://www.fda.gov/media/75191/download?attachment.

19 "Immune Response Rates for M-M-R®II (Measles, Mumps, and Rubella Virus Vaccine Live)." MerckVaccines.com, November 28, 2023. https://www.merckvaccines.com/mmr/efficacy/.

20 Hickman, Carole J., Terri B. Hyde, Sun Bae Sowers, Sara Mercader, Marcia McGrew, Nobia J. Williams, Judy A. Beeler, et al. "Laboratory Characterization of Measles Virus Infection in Previously Vaccinated and Unvaccinated Individuals." *Journal of Infectious Diseases* 204, no. suppl_1 (July 2011). https://doi.org/10.1093/infdis/jir106.

21 Haralambieva, Iana H., Richard B. Kennedy, Inna G. Ovsyannikova, Daniel J. Schaid, and Gregory A. Poland. "Current Perspectives in Assessing Humoral Immunity after Measles Vaccination." *Expert Review of Vaccines* 18, no. 1 (December 26, 2018): 75–87. https://doi.org/10.1080/14760584.2019.1559063.

22 Papania, Mark, Andrew L. Baughman, Susan Lee, James E. Cheek, William Atkinson, Stephen C. Redd, Kenneth Spitalny, Lyn Finelli, and Lauri Markowitz.

"Increased Susceptibility to Measles in Infants in the United States." *Pediatrics* 104, no. 5 (November 1, 1999). https://doi.org/10.1542/peds.104.5.e59.

23 Patel Manisha, Adria D. Lee, Susan B. Redd, Nakia S. Clemmons, Rebecca J. McNall, Amanda C. Cohn, and Paul A. Gastanaduy. "Increase in Measles Cases — United States, January 1–April 26, 2019." *Morbidity and Mortality Weekly Report* 68 (2019):402–404. DOI: http://dx.doi.org/10.15585/mmwr.mm6817e1.

24 Serres, Gaston De, Jean R. Joly, Micheline Fauvel, François Meyer, Benoit Mâsse, and Nicole Boulianne. "Passive Immunity against Measles during the First 8 Months of Life of Infants Born to Vaccinated Mothers or to Mothers Who Sustained Measles." *Vaccine* 15, no. 6–7 (April 1997): 620–23. https://doi.org/10.1016/s0264-410x(96)00283-6.

25 Fiebelkorn, Amy Parker, Laura A. Coleman, Edward A. Belongia, Sandra K. Freeman, Daphne York, Daoling Bi, Ashwin Kulkarni, et al. "Measles Virus Neutralizing Antibody Response, Cell-Mediated Immunity, and Immunoglobulin G Antibody Avidity before and after Receipt of a Third Dose of Measles, Mumps, and Rubella Vaccine in Young Adults." *Journal of Infectious Diseases* 213, no. 7 (November 23, 2015): 1115–23. https://doi.org/10.1093/infdis/jiv555.

26 Albonico, H.U., H.U. Bräker, and J. Hüsler. "Febrile Infectious Childhood Diseases in the History of Cancer Patients and Matched Control." *Medical Hypotheses* 51, no. 4 (October 1998): 315–20. https://doi.org/10.1016/s0306-9877(98)90055-x.

27 Sasco, Annie J., and Ralph S. Paffenbarger. "Measles Infection and Parkinson's Disease." *American Journal of Epidemiology* 122, no. 6 (December 1985): 1017–31. https://doi.org/10.1093/oxfordjournals.aje.a114183.

28 Montella, Maurizio, Luigino Dal Maso, Anna Crispo, Renato Talamini, Ettore Bidoli, Maria Grimaldi, Aldo Giudice, Antonio Pinto, and Silvia Franceschi. "Do Childhood Diseases Affect NHL and HL Risk? A Case-Control Study from Northern and Southern Italy." *Leukemia Research* 30, no. 8 (August 2006): 917–22. https://doi.org/10.1016/j.leukres.2005.11.020.

29 Alexander, F E., R F. Jarrett, D Lawrence, A A. Armstrong, J Freeland, D A. Gokhale, E Kane, G M. Taylor, D H. Wright, and R A. Cartwright. "Risk Factors for Hodgkin's Disease by Epstein-Barr Virus (EBV) Status: Prior Infection by EBV and Other Agents." *British Journal of Cancer* 82, no. 5 (March 2000): 1117–21. https://doi.org/10.1054/bjoc.1999.1049.

30 Aref, Sarah, Katharine Bailey, and Adele Fielding. "Measles to the Rescue: A Review of Oncolytic Measles Virus." *Viruses* 8, no. 10 (October 22, 2016): 294. https://doi.org/10.3390/v8100294.

31 "Mumps Complications." Centers for Disease Control and Prevention, March 8, 2021https://www.cdc.gov/mumps/about/complications.html.

32 "Measles, Mumps, and Rubella (MMR) Vaccination." Centers for Disease Control and Prevention, January 26, 2021. https://www.cdc.gov/vaccines/vpd/mmr/public/index.html.

33 Karimi, Faith. "Harvard Mumps Outbreak Grows; Dozens Infected." CNN, April 27, 2016. https://www.cnn.com/2016/04/27/health/harvard-university-mumps-outbreak/.

34 Rosario, Frank. "MUMPS Outbreak Hits Fordham University." *New York Post*, February 21, 2014. https://nypost.com/2014/02/21/mumps-outbreak-at-fordham-university/.

35 "8 Mumps Cases Reported at NJ College." ABC News, April 18, 2014. https://abcnews.go.com/Health/video/mumps-cases-reported-nj-college-23380716.

36 Lewnard, Joseph A., and Yonatan H. Grad. "Vaccine waning and mumps re-emergence in the United States." Science.org, March 21, 2018. Accessed January 25, 2024. https://www.science.org/doi/10.1126/scitranslmed.aao5945.

37 "Vaccine Excipient Summary." Centers for Disease Control and Prevention, November1,2021.https://www.cdc.gov/vaccines/pubs/pinkbook/rubella.html#secular-trends-in-US.

38 "Rubella in the United States." Centers for Disease Control and Prevention, November 14, 2023. https://www.cdc.gov/rubella/about/in-the-us.html#:

39 "Measles, Mumps, and Rubella (MMR) Vaccination." Centers for Disease Control and Prevention, January 26, 2021. https://www.cdc.gov/vaccines/vpd/mmr/public/index.html.

40 Merck Sharp & Dohme LLC. *Package Insert*. M-M-R II. U. S. Food and Drug Administration. August https://www.fda.gov/media/75191/download?attachment.

41 "Immune Response Rates for M-M-R®II (Measles, Mumps, and Rubella Virus Vaccine Live)." MerckVaccines.com, November 28, 2023. https://www.merckvaccines.com/mmr/efficacy/

42 Kung, Wan-Ju, Ching-Tang Shih, Yung-Luen Shih, Ling-Yao Liu, Chiou-Huey Wang, Ya-Wen Cheng, Hsueh-Chiao Liu, and Ching-Chiang Lin. "Faster Waning of the Rubella-specific Immune Response in Young Pregnant Women Immunized with MMR at 15 Months." *American Journal of Reproductive Immunology* 84, no. 4 (July 7, 2020). https://doi.org/10.1111/aji.13294.

Chapter 10

1 Gorda, Leada. "Measles in Alabama: What You Need to Know." AL.com, April 25, 2019. https://www.al.com/news/2019/04/measles-in-alabama-what-you-need-to-know-and-what-you-should-do.html.

2 Jain, Anjali, Jaclyn Marshall, Ami Buikema, Tim Bancroft, Jonathan P. Kelly, and Craig J. Newschaffer. "Autism Occurrence by MMR Vaccine Status among Us Children with Older Siblings with and without Autism." *JAMA* 313, no. 15 (April 21, 2015): 1534. https://doi.org/10.1001/jama.2015.3077.

3 Taylor, Luke E., Amy L. Swerdfeger, and Guy D. Eslick. "Vaccines Are Not Associated with Autism: An Evidence-Based Meta-Analysis of Case-Control and Cohort Studies." *Vaccine* 32, no. 29 (June 2014): 3623–29. https://doi.org/10.1016/j.vaccine.2014.04.085.

4 DeStefano, Frank, Tanya Karapurkar Bhasin, William W. Thompson, Marshalyn Yeargin-Allsopp, and Coleen Boyle. "Age at First Measles-Mumps-Rubella Vaccination in Children with Autism and School-Matched Control Subjects: A Population-Based Study in Metropolitan Atlanta." *Pediatrics* 113, no. 2 (February 1, 2004): 259–66. https://doi.org/10.1542/peds.113.2.259.

5 Smith, Nathaniel. "Statement of William W. Thompson, Ph.d., Regarding the 2004 Article Examining the Possibility of a Relationship between MMR Vaccine and Autism." Morgan Verkamp, July 19, 2023. https://morganverkamp.com/statement-of-william-w-thompson-ph-d-regarding-the-2004-article-examining-the-possibility-of-a-relationship-between-mmr-vaccine-and-autism/.

6 Hooker, Brian S. "Reanalysis of CDC Data on Autism Incidence and Time of First MMR Vaccination." *Journal of American Physicians and Surgeons.* 23, no. 4 (Winter 2018): 105-109. https://www.ncbi.nlm.nih.gov/pmc/articles/PMC4128611/.

7 Madsen, Kreesten Meldgaard, Anders Hviid, Mogens Vestergaard, Diana Schendel, Jan Wohlfahrt, Poul Thorsen, Jørn Olsen, and Mads Melbye. "A Population-Based Study of Measles, Mumps, and Rubella Vaccination and Autism." *New England Journal of Medicine* 347, no. 19 (November 7, 2002): 1477–82. https://doi.org/10.1056/nejmoa021134.

8 Remschmidt, Cornelius, Ole Wichmann, and Thomas Harder. "Frequency and Impact of Confounding by Indication and Healthy Vaccinee Bias in Observational Studies Assessing Influenza Vaccine Effectiveness: A Systematic Review." *BMC Infectious Diseases* 15, no. 1 (October 17, 2015). https://doi.org/10.1186/s12879-015-1154-y.

9 Ibid.

10 Ibid.

11 Ibid.

12 Hviid, Anders, Jørgen Vinsløv Hansen, Morten Frisch, and Mads Melbye. "Measles, Mumps, Rubella Vaccination and Autism." *Annals of Internal Medicine* 170, no. 8 (March 5, 2019): 513. https://doi.org/10.7326/m18-2101.

13 Ibid.

14 "Major New Vaccines Initiative Aims to Fight Deadly Airborne Infections." Novo Nordisk Fonden, December 20, 2023. https://novonordiskfonden.dk/en/news/major-new-vaccines-initiative-aims-to-fight-deadly-airborne-infections/#

15 Hviid, Anders, Jørgen Vinsløv Hansen, Morten Frisch, and Mads Melbye. "Measles, Mumps, Rubella Vaccination and Autism." *Annals of Internal Medicine* 170, no. 8 (March 5, 2019): 513. https://doi.org/10.7326/m18-2101.

16 Mawson, Anthony R, Azad Bhuiyan, Binu Jacob, and Brian D. Ray. "Preterm Birth, Vaccination and Neurodevelopmental Disorders: A Cross-Sectional Study of 6- to 12-Year-Old Vaccinated and Unvaccinated Children." *Journal of Translational Science* 3, no. 3 (2017). https://doi.org/10.15761/jts.1000187.

17 Ibid.

18 DeLong, Gayle. "A Positive Association Found between Autism Prevalence and Childhood Vaccination Uptake across the U.S. Population." *Journal of Toxicology and Environmental Health*, Part A 74, no. 14 (July 15, 2011): 903–16. https://doi.org/10.1080/15287394.2011.573736.

19 Singh, Vijendra K., Sheren X. Lin, Elizabeth Newell, and Courtney Nelson. "Abnormal Measles-Mumps-Rubella Antibodies and CNS Autoimmunity in Children with Autism." *Journal of Biomedical Science* 9, no. 4 (July 2002): 359–64. https://doi.org/10.1007/bf02256592.

20 Singh, Vijendra K., and Ryan L. Jensen. "Elevated Levels of Measles Antibodies in Children with Autism." *Pediatric Neurology* 28, no. 4 (April 2003): 292–94. https://doi.org/10.1016/s0887-8994(02)00627-6.

21 Weibel, Robert E., Vito Caserta, David E. Benor, and Geoffrey Evans. "Acute Encephalopathy Followed by Permanent Brain Injury or Death Associated with Further Attenuated Measles Vaccines: A Review of Claims Submitted to the National Vaccine Injury Compensation Program." *Pediatrics* 101, no. 3 (March 1, 1998): 383–87. https://doi.org/10.1542/peds.101.3.383.

22 Ibid.

23 "Inbrief: The Science of Early Childhood Development." Center on the Developing Child at Harvard University, October 29, 2020. https://developingchild.harvard.edu/resources/inbrief-science-of-ecd/.

Chapter 11

1 "Varicella Vaccine Recommendations." Centers for Disease Control and Prevention, April 28, 2021. https://www.cdc.gov/vaccines/vpd/varicella/hcp/recommendations.html.

2 Merck Sharp & Dohme LLC. *Package Insert: VARIVAX.* Food and Drug Administration (FDA), August, 2023. https://www.fda.gov/media/76000/download.

3 "Vaccine Excipient Summary." Centers for Disease Control and Prevention, November 1, 2021. https://www.cdc.gov/vaccines/pubs/pinkbook/downloads/appendices/b/excipient-table-2.pdf.

4 Ibid.

5 "Varicella Vaccine Recommendations." Centers for Disease Control and Prevention, April 28, 2021. https://www.cdc.gov/vaccines/vpd/varicella/hcp/recommendations.html.

6 Lee, Young Hwa, Young June Choe, Kwan Hong, Yoonsun Yoon, and Yun-Kyung Kim. "The Protective Effectiveness of 2-Dose Varicella Vaccination in Children in Korea: A Case-Control Study." *Pediatric Infectious Disease Journal* 42, no. 8 (May 26, 2023): 719–22. https://doi.org/10.1097/inf.0000000000003958.

7 Weinmann, Sheila, Allison L. Naleway, Padma Koppolu, Roger Baxter, Edward A. Belongia, Simon J. Hambidge, Stephanie A. Irving, et al. "Incidence of Herpes Zoster among Children: 2003–2014." *Pediatrics* 144, no. 1 (July 1, 2019). https://doi.org/10.1542/peds.2018-2917.

8 Merck Sharp & Dohme LLC. *Product Insert: VARIVAX.* August, 2023. Food and Drug Administration. https://www.fda.gov/media/76000/download.

9 "About the Varicella Vaccine." Centers for Disease Control and Prevention, April 28, 2021. https://www.cdc.gov/vaccines/vpd/varicella/hcp/about-vaccine.html.

10 Merck Sharp & Dohme LLC. *Product Insert: VARIVAX.* U.S. Food and Drug Administration. August, 2023. https://www.fda.gov/media/76000/download.

11 Vázquez, Marietta. "Effectiveness over Time of Varicella Vaccine." *JAMA* 291, no. 7 (February 18, 2004): 851. https://doi.org/10.1001/jama.291.7.851.

12 "Clinical Overview of Herpes Zoster (Shingles)." Centers for Disease Control and Prevention, May 10, 2023. https://www.cdc.gov/shingles/hcp/clinical-overview.html.

13 Goldman, G.S., and P.G. King. "Review of the United States Universal Varicella Vaccination Program: Herpes Zoster Incidence Rates, Cost-Effectiveness, and Vaccine Efficacy Based Primarily on the Antelope Valley Varicella Active Surveillance Project Data." *Vaccine* 31, no. 13 (March 2013): 1680–94. https://doi.org/10.1016/j.vaccine.2012.05.050.

14 Yawn, Barbara P., Robbin F. Itzler, Peter C. Wollan, James M. Pellissier, Lina S. Sy, and Patricia Saddier. "Health Care Utilization and Cost Burden of Herpes Zoster in a Community Population." *Mayo Clinic Proceedings* 84, no. 9 (September 2009): 787–94. https://doi.org/10.4065/84.9.787.

15 Harpaz, Rafael, and Jessica W Leung. "The Epidemiology of Herpes Zoster in the United States during the Era of Varicella and Herpes Zoster Vaccines: Changing Patterns among Older Adults." *Clinical Infectious Diseases* 69, no. 2 (November 29, 2018): 341–44. https://doi.org/10.1093/cid/ciy953.

16 Brisson, M., N.J. Gay, W.J. Edmunds, and N.J. Andrews. "Exposure to Varicella Boosts Immunity to Herpes-Zoster: Implications for Mass Vaccination against Chickenpox." *Vaccine* 20, no. 19–20 (June 2002): 2500–2507. https://doi.org/10.1016/s0264-410x(02)00180-9.

17 Ibid.

Chapter 12

1 "Haemophilus Influenzae: Causes, How It Spreads, and People at Increased Risk." Centers for Disease Control and Prevention, March 4, 2022. https://www.cdc.gov/hi-disease/about/causes-transmission.html.

2 "Pinkbook: Haemophilus Influenzae (Hib)." Centers for Disease Control and Prevention, August 18, 2021. https://www.cdc.gov/vaccines/pubs/pinkbook/hib.html.

3 "For Clinicians: Haemophilus Influenzae." Centers for Disease Control and Prevention, March 4, 2022. https://www.cdc.gov/hi-disease/clinicians.html.

4 "Haemophilus Influenzae: Types of Infection." Centers for Disease Control and Prevention, March 4, 2022https://cdc.gov/hi-disease/about/types-infection.html.

5 "About Hib Vaccine (Haemophilus Influenzae Type B Vaccine)." Centers for Disease Control and Prevention, April 13, 2021. https://www.cdc.gov/vaccines/vpd/hib/hcp/about-vaccine.html.

6 Ibid.

7 "Vaccine Excipient Summary." Centers for Disease Control and Prevention, November 1, 2021. https://www.cdc.gov/vaccines/pubs/pinkbook/downloads/appendices/b/excipient-table-2.pdf.

8 Ibid.

9 428. Merck & Co. Inc. *Package Insert: LIQUID PEDVAXHIB*. Food and Drug Administration. 1998. https://www.fda.gov/media/80438/download?attachment.

10 Soeters, Heidi M, Amy Blain, Tracy Pondo, Brooke Doman, Monica M Farley, Lee H Harrison, Ruth Lynfield, et al. "Current Epidemiology and Trends in Invasive Haemophilus Influenzae Disease—United States, 2009–2015." *Clinical Infectious Diseases* 67, no. 6 (March 2, 2018): 881–89. https://doi.org/10.1093/cid/ciy187.

11 "Hib Vaccination: What Everyone Should Know." Centers for Disease Control and Prevention, April 13, 2021. https://www.cdc.gov/vaccines/vpd/hib/public/index.html.

12 Ibid.

Chapter 13

1 "Hepatitis A Vaccines for Children." Centers for Disease Control and Prevention, August 2, 2019. https://www.cdc.gov/vaccines/parents/diseases/hepa.html.

2 "Hepatitis A—Faqs, Statistics, Data, & Guidelines." Centers for Disease Control and Prevention, June 22, 2020. https://www.cdc.gov/hepatitis/hav/index.htm.

3 "What Is Hepatitis A—FAQ." Centers for Disease Control and Prevention, July 28, 2020. https://www.cdc.gov/hepatitis/hav/afaq.htm#D2.

4 "Hepatitis A Vaccine Information Statement." Centers for Disease Control and Prevention, October 15, 2021. https://www.cdc.gov/vaccines/hcp/vis/vis-statements/hep-a.html.

5 "Hepatitis A Q&as for Health Professionals." Centers for Disease Control and Prevention, September 27, 2023. https://www.cdc.gov/hepatitis/hav/havfaq.htm.

6 "Hepatitis A Vaccine Information Statement." Centers for Disease Control and Prevention, October 15, 2021. https://www.cdc.gov/vaccines/hcp/vis/vis-statements/hep-a.html.

7 "Pinkbook: Hepatitis A." Centers for Disease Control and Prevention, August 18, 2021. https://www.cdc.gov/vaccines/pubs/pinkbook/hepa.html.

8 Ibid.

9 GlaxoSmithKline Biologicals. *Product Insert: HAVRIX.* U.S. Food and Drug Administration.XXXX.https://www.fda.gov/media/119388/download?attachment

10 Ibid.

11 Fulgenzi, Alessandro, Daniele Vietti, and Maria Elena Ferrero. "Aluminium Involvement in Neurotoxicity." *BioMed Research International* 2014 (2014): 1–5. https://doi.org/10.1155/2014/758323.

12 Merck & Co., Inc. *Package Insert: VAQTA.* Food and Drug Administration (FDA), 20XX. https://www.fda.gov/media/74519/download?attachment.

13 Ibid.

14 Mold, Matthew, Caroline Linhart, Johana Gómez-Ramírez, Andrés Villegas-Lanau, and Christopher Exley. "Aluminum and Amyloid-β in Familial Alzheimer's Disease." *Journal of Alzheimer's Disease* 73, no. 4 (February 18, 2020): 1627–35. https://doi.org/10.3233/jad-191140.

15 Mold, Matthew, Dorcas Umar, Andrew King, and Christopher Exley. "Aluminium in Brain Tissue in Autism." *Journal of Trace Elements in Medicine and Biology* 46 (March 2018): 76–82. https://doi.org/10.1016/j.jtemb.2017.11.012.

16 Exley, Christopher, and Elizabeth Clarkson. "Aluminium in Human Brain Tissue from Donors without Neurodegenerative Disease: A Comparison with Alzheimer's Disease, Multiple Sclerosis and Autism." *Scientific Reports* 10, no. 1 (May 8, 2020). https://doi.org/10.1038/s41598-020-64734-6.

17 "Pinkbook: Hepatitis A." Centers for Disease Control and Prevention, August 18, 2021 https://www.cdc.gov/vaccines/pubs/pinkbook/hepa.html#vaccines.

Chapter 14

1 "What Is Polio?" Centers for Disease Control and Prevention, August 11, 2022. https://www.cdc.gov/polio/what-is-polio/index.htm.

2 "Why CDC Is Working to End Polio Globally." Centers for Disease Control and Prevention, June 28, 2023. https://www.cdc.gov/polio/why-are-we-involved/index.htm.

3 Ibid.

4 "What Is Polio?" Centers for Disease Control and Prevention, August 11, 2022. https://www.cdc.gov/polio/what-is-polio/index.htm.

5 "Post-Polio Syndrome." Centers for Disease Control and Prevention, September 23, 2021. https://www.cdc.gov/polio/what-is-polio/pps.html.

6 "Polio + Prevention." Global Polio Eradication Initiative. Accessed January 25, 2024. https://polioeradication.org/polio-today/polio-prevention/#.

7 "Polio Vaccine Composition, Dosage, Administration, and Administration Errors." Centers for Disease Control and Prevention, August 8, 2022. https://www.cdc.gov/vaccines/vpd/polio/hcp/composition-dosage-administration.html.

8 Selected Discontinued U.S. Vaccines. Centers for Disease Control and Prevention. Accessed January 26, 2024. https://www.cdc.gov/vaccines/pubs/pinkbook/downloads/appendices/b/discontinued_vaccines.pdf.

9 "Vaccine Excipient Summary." Centers for Disease Control and Prevention, November 1, 2021. https://www.cdc.gov/vaccines/pubs/pinkbook/downloads/appendices/b/excipient-table-2.pdf.

10 Ibid.

11 "Contraindications and Precautions for Polio Vaccination." Centers for Disease Control and Prevention, August 8, 2022. https://www.cdc.gov/vaccines/vpd/polio/hcp/contraindications-precautions.html.

12 Institute of Medicine (US) Vaccine Safety Committee. "Adverse Events Associated with Childhood Vaccines: Evidence Bearing on Causality." Edited by Kathleen R. Stratton, Cynthia J. Howe, and Richard B. Johnston. National Academies Press (US), 1994. https://doi.org/DOI:10.17226/2138.

13 Wallace, Gregory S., Aaron T. Curns, William C. Weldon, and M. Steven Oberste. "Seroprevalence of Poliovirus Antibodies in the United States Population, 2009–2010." *BMC Public Health* 16, no. 1 (August 5, 2016). https://doi.org/10.1186/s12889-016-3386-1.

14 Spaendonck, M. A. van, P. M. Oostvogel, A. M. van Loon, J. K. van Wijngaarden, and D. Kromhout. "Circulation of Poliovirus during the Poliomyelitis Outbreak in the Netherlands in 1992-1993." *American Journal of Epidemiology* 143, no. 9 (May 1, 1996): 929–35. https://doi.org/10.1093/oxfordjournals.aje.a008836.

Chapter 15

1 Kim, Gyu-Lee, Seung-Han Seon, and Dong-Kwon Rhee. "Pneumonia and Streptococcus Pneumoniae Vaccine." *Archives of Pharmacal Research* 40, no. 8 (July 22, 2017): 885–93. https://doi.org/10.1007/s12272-017-0933-y.

2 American Lung Association. "What Causes Pneumonia?" August 3, 2023. https://www.lung.org/lung-health-diseases/lung-disease-lookup/pneumonia/what-causes-pneumonia.

3 "Pneumococcal Disease: Risk Factors and How It Spreads." Centers for Disease Control and Prevention. September 21, 2023. https://www.cdc.gov/pneumococcal/about/risk-transmission.html.

4 Ibid.

5 "Symptoms and Complications of Pneumococcal Disease." Centers for Disease Control and Prevention. May 18, 2022. https://www.cdc.gov/pneumococcal/about/symptoms-complications.html.

6 "Diagnosis and Treatment of Pneumococcal Disease." Centers for Disease Control and Prevention. September 1, 2020. https://www.cdc.gov/pneumococcal/about/diagnosis-treatment.html.

7 "Pneumococcal Disease Surveillance Reporting and Trends." Centers for Disease Control and Prevention. September 21, 2023. https://www.cdc.gov/pneumococcal/surveillance.html.

8 "Administering Pneumococcal Vaccine: For Prevention." Centers for Disease Control and Prevention. September 21, 2023. https://www.cdc.gov/vaccines/vpd/pneumo/hcp/administering-vaccine.html.

9 "Vaccine Excipient Summary." Centers for Disease Control and Prevention, November 1, 2021. https://www.cdc.gov/vaccines/pubs/pinkbook/downloads/appendices/b/excipient-table-2.pdf.

10 Ibid.

11 "Administering Pneumococcal Vaccine: For Prevention." for Disease Control and Prevention.September 21, 2023. https://www.cdc.gov/vaccines/vpd/pneumo/hcp/administering-vaccine.html.

12 "Pneumococcal Vaccination: What Everyone Should Know." Centers for Disease Control and Prevention. September 21, 2023. https://www.cdc.gov/vaccines/vpd/pneumo/public/index.html.

13 Abbasi, Jennifer. "The Flawed Science of Antibody Testing for SARS-COV-2 Immunity." *JAMA* 326, no. 18 (November 9, 2021): 1781. https://jamanetwork.com/journals/jama/fullarticle/2785530.

14 Food and Drug Administration. "Package Insert—PREVNAR 20." Food and Drug Administration (FDA), 202X. https://www.fda.gov/media/149987/download?attachment.

15 Ibid.

16 Food and Drug Administration. "Package Insert—PNEUMOVAX 23." Food and Drug Administration (FDA), April 2021. https://www.fda.gov/media/80547/download?attachment.

17 Galanis, Ilias, Ann Lindstrand, Jessica Darenberg, Sarah Browall, Priyanka Nannapaneni, Karin Sjöström, Eva Morfeldt, et al. "Effects of PCV7 and

PCV13 on Invasive Pneumococcal Disease and Carriage in Stockholm, Sweden." *The European Respiratory Journal* 47, no. 4 (January 21, 2016): 1208–18. https://pubmed.ncbi.nlm.nih.gov/26797033/.

18 Ibid.

Chapter 16

1 "Transmission of Rotavirus." Centers for Disease Control and Prevention, March 26, 2021. https://www.cdc.gov/rotavirus/about/transmission.html.

2 "Rotavirus in the U.S." Centers for Disease Control and Prevention, March 26, 2021. https://www.cdc.gov/rotavirus/surveillance.html.

3 "Treatment of Rotavirus." Centers for Disease Control and Prevention, March 26, 2021. https://www.cdc.gov/rotavirus/about/treatment.html.

4 "Rotavirus Vaccines." Centers for Disease Control and Prevention, March 26, 2021. https://www.cdc.gov/rotavirus/vaccination.html.

5 "Vaccine Excipient Summary." Centers for Disease Control and Prevention, November 1, 2021. https://www.cdc.gov/vaccines/pubs/pinkbook/downloads/appendices/b/excipient-table-2.pdf.

6 "Administering the Rotavirus Vaccine." Centers for Disease Control and Prevention, March 25, 2021. https://www.cdc.gov/vaccines/vpd/rotavirus/hcp/administering-vaccine.html.

7 "Rotavirus Vaccine Recommendations: For Providers." Centers for Disease Control and Prevention, March 25, 2021. https://www.cdc.gov/vaccines/vpd/rotavirus/hcp/recommendations.html.

8 Parashar, Umesh D., Erik G. Hummelman, Joseph S. Bresee, Mark A. Miller, and Roger I. Glass. "Global Illness and Deaths Caused by Rotavirus Disease in Children." *Emerging Infectious Diseases* 9, no. 5 (May 2003): 565–72. https://doi.org/10.3201/eid0905.020562.

9 Ma, Liyuan, Antoine C. El Khoury, and Robbin F. Itzler. "The Burden of Rotavirus Hospitalizations among Medicaid and Non-Medicaid Children Younger than 5 Years Old." *American Journal of Public Health* 99, no. S2 (October 2009). https://doi.org/10.2105/ajph.2008.148494.

10 GlaxoSmithKline Biologicals. *Package Insert: ROTARIX*. Food and Drug Administration (FDA), 20XX. https://www.fda.gov/media/75726/download.

11 "About Rotavirus Vaccine: For Providers." Centers for Disease Control and Prevention, March 25, 2021.https://www.cdc.gov/vaccines/vpd/rotavirus/hcp/about-vaccine.html#:

12 Baker, Julia M., Jacqueline E. Tate, Claudia A. Steiner, Michael J. Haber, Umesh D. Parashar, and Benjamin A. Lopman. "Longer-Term Direct and Indirect Effects of Infant Rotavirus Vaccination across All Ages in the United States in 2000–2013: Analysis of a Large Hospital Discharge Data Set." *Clinical Infectious Diseases* 68, no. 6 (July 18, 2018): 976–83. https://doi.org/10.1093/cid/ciy580.

13 GlaxoSmithKline Biologicals. *Package Insert: ROTARIX.* Food and Drug Administration (FDA), 20XX. https://www.fda.gov/media/75726/download.

14 Ibid.
15 Ibid.
16 "ECDC Expert opinion on rotavirus vaccination in infancy." European Centre for Disease Prevention and Control. Stockholm: ECDC; 2017. https://www.ecdc.europa.eu/sites/default/files/documents/rotavirus-vaccination-expert%20opinion-september-2017.pdf.
17 Ibid.
18 Ibid.

Chapter 17

1 Fichera, Angelo. "No, Covid-19 Vaccines Aren't Gene Therapy." AP News, December 23, 2022. https://apnews.com/article/fact-check-covid-vaccines-gene-therapy-806280914802.
2 "Unlocking the Power of Our Body's Protein Factory." Pfizer. June, 2022. https://www.pfizer.com/news/behind-the-science/unlocking-power-our-bodys-protein-factory#.
3 Thucydides. 1963. *History of the Peloponnesian War.* Translated by Rex Warner. Penguin Classics. London, England: Penguin Classics.
4 Dolgin, Elie. "Self-Copying RNA Vaccine Wins First Full Approval: What's Next?" Nature News, December 6, 2023. https://www.nature.com/articles/d41586-023-03859-w.
5 Constantino, Annika Kim. "New Covid Vaccines Are Coming to the U.S. This Fall, but Uptake May Be Low—Here's Why." CNBC, July 29, 2023. https://www.cnbc.com/2023/07/29/covid-vaccine-what-uptake-of-new-shots-could-look-like.html.
6 Constantino, Annika Kim. "Pfizer's Combination Covid, Flu Vaccine Will Move to Final-Stage Trial after Positive Data." CNBC, October 26, 2023. https://www.cnbc.com/2023/10/26/pfizer-combination-covid-flu-vaccine-shows-positive-trial-data.html.
7 "Harnessing the Potential of mRNA." Pfizer. November 18, 2020. Accessed January 25, 2024. https://www.pfizer.com/science/innovation/mrna-technology.
8 Röltgen, Katharina, Sandra C.A. Nielsen, Oscar Silva, Sheren F. Younes, Maxim Zaslavsky, Cristina Costales, Fan Yang, et al. "Immune Imprinting, Breadth of Variant Recognition, and Germinal Center Response in Human SARS-COV-2 Infection and Vaccination." *Cell* 185, no. 6 (March 2022). https://doi.org/10.1016/j.cell.2022.01.018.
9 Brogna, Carlo, Simone Cristoni, Giuliano Marino, Luigi Montano, Valentina Viduto, Mark Fabrowski, Gennaro Lettieri, and Marina Piscopo. "Detection of Recombinant Spike Protein in the Blood of Individuals Vaccinated against Sars-cov-2: Possible Molecular Mechanisms." *PROTEOMICS—Clinical Applications* 17, no. 6 (August 31, 2023). https://doi.org/10.1002/prca.202300048.
10 Mulroney, Thomas E., Tuija Pöyry, Juan Carlos Yam-Puc, Maria Rust, Robert F. Harvey, Lajos Kalmar, Emily Horner, et al. "N1-Methylpseudouridylation of Mrna Causes +1 Ribosomal Frameshifting." *Nature* 625, no. 7993 (December 6, 2023): 189–94. https://doi.org/10.1038/s41586-023-06800-3.

11 Ibid.
12 Malone, Robert, Gwendolyn Kull, Jeffrey A. Tucker, Debbie Lerman, Brownstone Institute, Ramesh Thakur, and Rebekah Barnett. "The Delights of the Pfizer/Moderna Catfight–Brownstone Institute." Brownstone Institute, September 3, 2023. https://brownstone.org/articles/delights-of-the-pfizer-moderna-catfight/.
13 Garde, Damian. "Ego, Ambition, and Turmoil: Inside One of Biotech's Most Secretive Startups." STAT, September 13, 2016. https://www.statnews.com/2016/09/13/moderna-therapeutics-biotech-mrna/.
14 Bitounis, Dimitrios, Eric Jacquinet, Maximillian A. Rogers, and Mansoor M. Amiji. "Strategies to Reduce the Risks of Mrna Drug and Vaccine Toxicity." *Nature Reviews Drug Discovery*, January 23, 2024.
15 Najahi-Missaoui, Wided, Robert D. Arnold, and Brian S. Cummings. "Safe Nanoparticles: Are We There Yet?" *International Journal of Molecular Sciences* 22, no. 1 (December 31, 2020): 385. https://doi.org/10.3390/ijms22010385.
16 Hou, Xucheng, Tal Zaks, Robert Langer, and Yizhou Dong. "Lipid Nanoparticles for Mrna Delivery." *Nature Reviews Materials* 6, no. 12 (August 10, 2021): 1078–94. https://doi.org/10.1038/s41578-021-00358-0.
17 La-Beck, Ninh M., Md. Rakibul Islam, and Maciej M. Markiewski. "Nanoparticle-Induced Complement Activation: Implications for Cancer Nanomedicine." Frontiers, November 23, 2020. https://www.frontiersin.org/articles/10.3389/fimmu.2020.603039/full.
18 Ihle-Hansen, Håkon, Håkon Bøås, German Tapia, Guri Hagberg, Hege Ihle-Hansen, Jacob Dag Berild, Randi Selmer, Øystein Karlstad, Hanne Løvdal Gulseth, and Inger Ariansen. "Stroke after SARS-COV-2 Mrna Vaccine: A Nationwide Registry Study." *Stroke* 54, no. 5 (May 2023). https://doi.org/10.1161/strokeaha.122.040430.
19 Alami, Abdallah, Daniel Krewski, Nawal Farhat, Donald Mattison, Kumanan Wilson, Christopher A. Gravel, Patrick J. Farrell, et al. "Risk of Myocarditis and Pericarditis in Mrna COVID-19-Vaccinated and Unvaccinated Populations: A Systematic Review and Meta-Analysis." *BMJ Open* 13, no. 6 (June 2023). https://doi.org/10.1136/bmjopen-2022-065687.
20 Oster, Matthew E., David K. Shay, John R. Su, Julianne Gee, C. Buddy Creech, Karen R. Broder, Kathryn Edwards, et al. "Myocarditis Cases Reported after Mrna-Based COVID-19 Vaccination in the US from December 2020 to August 2021." *JAMA* 327, no. 4 (January 25, 2022): 331. https://doi.org/10.1001/jama.2021.24110.
21 Brown, Amanda. "Pfizer's Own Study Finds Nanoparticles in Covid Vaccines Enter Organs." *Western Standard*. May 11, 2022. https://www.westernstandard.news/business/pfizer-s-own-study-finds-nanoparticles-in-covid-vaccines-enter-organs/article_5b3955f6-d146-11ec-a272-cf3264db392b.html.
22 Zhou, Zhiqian, Julia Barrett, and Xuan He. "Immune Imprinting and Implications for COVID-19." *Vaccines* 11, no. 4 (April 20, 2023): 875. https://doi.org/10.3390/vaccines11040875.
23 Shrestha, Nabin K., Patrick C. Burke, Amy S. Nowacki, James F. Simon, Amanda Hagen, and Steven M. Gordon. "Effectiveness of the coronavirus disease 2019

(COVID-19) bivalent vaccine," December 19, 2022. https://doi.org/10.1101/2022.12.17.22283625.

Chapter 18

1 Carlson, Robert H. "HPV Vaccine, Now FDA-Approved, Shown to Protect against Vaginal, Vulvar Intraepithelial Neoplasias." *Oncology Times* Supplement (August 2006): 2–4. https://doi.org/10.1097/01.cot.0000316086.11194.af.

2 "HPV Vaccine." Centers for Disease Control and Prevention, August 16, 2023. https://www.cdc.gov/hpv/parents/vaccine-for-hpv.html.

3 Ibid.

4 Luria L, Cardoza-Favarato G. "Human Papillomavirus." StatPearls [Internet]. Treasure Island, FL. StatPearls Publishing. (January 2024). https://www.ncbi.nlm.nih.gov/books/NBK448132/

5 Anna Szymonowicz, Klaudia, and Junjie Chen. "Biological and Clinical Aspects of HPV-Related Cancers." *Cancer Biology and Medicine* 17, no. 4 (2020): 864–78. https://doi.org/10.20892/j.issn.2095-3941.2020.0370.

6 Erkinovich, Nazarov Jalolitdin Sulton. "HPV—Relevance, Oncogenesis and Diagnosis (A Review)". *European Journal of Innovation in Nonformal Education* 3, no. 1 (2023):129-34. https://www.inovatus.es/index.php/ejine/article/view/1426.

7 "HPV and Cancer." National Cancer Institute. Accessed January 25, 2024. https://www.cancer.gov/about-cancer/causes-prevention/risk/infectious-agents/hpv-and-cancer.

8 Ibid.

9 Ibid.

10 "HPV-Associated Cancer Diagnosis by Age." Centers for Disease Control and Prevention, September 12, 2023. https://www.cdc.gov/cancer/hpv/statistics/age.htm.

11 Arbyn, Marc, Elisabete Weiderpass, Laia Bruni, Silvia de Sanjosé, Mona Saraiya, Jacques Ferlay, and Freddie Bray. "Estimates of Incidence and Mortality of Cervical Cancer in 2018: A Worldwide Analysis." *The Lancet Global Health* 8, no. 2 (February 2020). https://doi.org/10.1016/s2214-109x(19)30482-6.

12 Ibid.

13 "Cancer of the Cervix Uteri—Cancer Stat Facts." SEER. Accessed January 25, 2024. https://seer.cancer.gov/statfacts/html/cervix.html.

14 The Future II Study Group. "Quadrivalent Vaccine against Human Papillomavirus to Prevent High-Grade Cervical Lesions." *New England Journal of Medicine* 356, no. 19 (May 10, 2007): 1915–27. https://doi.org/10.1056/nejmoa061741.

15 Merck Sharp & Dohme LLC. *GARDASIL*. Food and Drug Administration. April, 2023. https://www.fda.gov/media/90064/download?attachment.

16 Vink, Margaretha A., Johannes A. Bogaards, Folkert J. van Kemenade, Hester E. de Melker, Chris J. Meijer, and Johannes Berkhof. "Clinical Progression of High-Grade Cervical Intraepithelial Neoplasia: Estimating the Time to Preclinical Cervical Cancer from Doubly Censored National Registry Data." *American Journal of Epidemiology* 178, no. 7 (July 28, 2013): 1161–69. https://doi.org/10.1093/aje/kwt077.

17 Burnett, Tatnai. "Do Atypical Cells Usually Mean Cancer?" Mayo Clinic, September 16, 2022. https://www.mayoclinic.org/diseases-conditions/cancer/expert-answers/atypical-cells/faq-20058493.

18 Vink, Margaretha A., Johannes A. Bogaards, Folkert J. van Kemenade, Hester E. de Melker, Chris J. Meijer, and Johannes Berkhof. "Clinical Progression of High-Grade Cervical Intraepithelial Neoplasia: Estimating the Time to Preclinical Cervical Cancer from Doubly Censored National Registry Data." *American Journal of Epidemiology* 178, no. 7 (July 28, 2013): 1161–69. https://doi.org/10.1093/aje/kwt077.

19 "Abnormal Pap Smear Follow-Up." Roswell Park Comprehensive Cancer Center. Accessed January 25, 2024. https://www.roswellpark.org/cancertalk/201811/abnormal-pap-smear-follow.

20 Baden, Lindsey R., Gregory D. Curfman, Stephen Morrissey, and Jeffrey M. Drazen. "Human Papillomavirus Vaccine—Opportunity and Challenge." *New England Journal of Medicine* 356, no. 19 (May 10, 2007): 1990–91. https://doi.org/10.1056/nejme078088.

21 Slade, Barbara A. "Postlicensure Safety Surveillance for Quadrivalent Human Papillomavirus Recombinant Vaccine." *JAMA* 302, no. 7 (August 19, 2009): 750. https://doi.org/10.1001/jama.2009.1201.

22 Ibid.

23 "HPV Vaccine Safety and Effectiveness." Centers for Disease Control and Prevention, November 16, 2021. https://www.cdc.gov/vaccines/vpd/hpv/hcp/safety-effectiveness.html.

24 Ibid.

25 Ibid.

26 Merck Sharp & Dohme LLC. *GARDASIL.* Food and Drug Administration. April, 2023. https://www.fda.gov/media/90064/download?attachment.

27 Hviid, A., H. Svanström, N. M. Scheller, O. Grönlund, B. Pasternak, and L. Arnheim-Dahlström. "Human Papillomavirus Vaccination of Adult Women and Risk of Autoimmune and Neurological Diseases." *Journal of Internal Medicine* 283, no. 2 (October 18, 2017): 154–65. https://doi.org/10.1111/joim.12694.

28 Little, Deirdre Therese, and Harvey Rodrick Ward. "Adolescent Premature Ovarian Insufficiency Following Human Papillomavirus Vaccination." *Journal of Investigative Medicine High Impact Case Reports* 2, no. 4 (October 1, 2014) https://doi.org/10.1177/2324709614556129.

29 Segal, Yahel, and Yehuda Shoenfeld. "Vaccine-Induced Autoimmunity: The Role of Molecular Mimicry and Immune Crossreaction." *Cellular & Molecular Immunology* 15, no. 6 (March 5, 2018): 586–94. https://doi.org/10.1038/cmi.2017.151.

30 Ivette Maldonado, Nicolas Rodríguez Niño, et al. "Evaluation of the safety profile of the quadrivalent vaccine against human papillomavirus in the risk of developing autoimmune, neurological, and hematological diseases in adolescent women in Colombia." Vaccine. Published online. (March 7, 2024). https://www.sciencedirect.com/science/article/pii/S0264410X24002639.

31 Merck Sharp & Dohme LLC. *GARDASIL.* Food and Drug Administration. April, 2023. https://www.fda.gov/media/90064/download?attachment.

32 Ibid.

33 Martínez-Lavín, Manuel. "HPV Vaccination Syndrome: A Clinical Mirage, or a New Tragic Fibromyalgia Model." *Reumatología Clínica* (English Edition) 14, no. 4 (July 2018): 211–14. https://doi.org/10.1016/j.reumae.2018.01.001.

34 Merck Sharp & Dohme LLC. *GARDASIL.* Food and Drug Administration. April, 2023. https://www.fda.gov/media/90064/download?attachment.

35 Shaw, Christopher A., and Michael S. Petrik. "Aluminum Hydroxide Injections Lead to Motor Deficits and Motor Neuron Degeneration." *Journal of Inorganic Biochemistry* 103, no. 11 (November 2009): 1555–62. https://doi.org/10.1016/j.jinorgbio.2009.05.019.

36 Shaw, C. A., and L. Tomljenovic. "Aluminum in the Central Nervous System (CNS): Toxicity in Humans and Animals, Vaccine Adjuvants, and Autoimmunity." *Immunologic Research* 56, no. 2–3 (April 23, 2013): 304–16. https://doi.org/10.1007/s12026-013-8403-1.

37 Exley, Christopher, and Elizabeth Clarkson. "Aluminium in Human Brain Tissue from Donors without Neurodegenerative Disease: A Comparison with Alzheimer's Disease, Multiple Sclerosis and Autism." *Scientific Reports* 10, no. 1 (May 8, 2020). https://doi.org/10.1038/s41598-020-64734-6.

38 Mehlsen, Jesper, Louise Brinth, Kirsten Pors, Kim Varming, Gerd Wallukat, and Rikke Katrine Olsen. "Autoimmunity in Patients Reporting Long-Term Complications after Exposure to Human Papilloma Virus Vaccination." *Journal of Autoimmunity* 133 (December 2022): 102921. https://doi.org/10.1016/j.jaut.2022.102921.

39 Ibid.

40 Ibid.

41 Lippman, Abby, Madeline Boscoe, and Carol Scurfield. "Do you approve of spending $300 million on HPV vaccination?: No." *Canadian family physician Medecin de famille canadien*, 54, no. 2, (2008) 175–181. https://www.ncbi.nlm.nih.gov/pmc/articles/PMC2278297/.

42 "List of grants for research to increase uptake of HPV vaccines." Children's Health Defense. Accessed January 26, 2024. https://childrenshealthdefense.org/wp-content/uploads/02-20-2020-Facts-about-HPV.pdf.

43 "Gavi Board Meeting, 7-8 December 2022." Gavi, The Vaccine Alliance. December, 2022. Accessed January 25, 2024. https://www.gavi.org/governance/gavi-board/minutes/7-8-december-2022.

44 "About Our Alliance." Gavi, The Vaccine Alliance. Accessed January 25, 2024. https://www.gavi.org/our-alliance/about.

45 Pharmacovigilance Risk Assessment Committee (PRAC). "Assessment Report: Human Papillomavirus (HPV) Vaccines," November 11, 2015. https://www.ema.europa.eu/en/documents/referral/hpv-vaccines-article-20-procedure-assessment-report_en.pdf.

46 Ibid.

47 Abouelella, Dina K., Julia E. Canick, Justin M. Barnes, Rebecca L. Rohde, Tammara L. Watts, Eric Adjei Boakye, and Nosayaba Osazuwa-Peters. "Human Papillomavirus Vaccine Uptake among Teens before and during the Covid-19 Pandemic in the United States." *Human Vaccines & Immunotherapeutics* 18, no. 7 (December 9, 2022). https://doi.org/10.1080/21645515.2022.2148825.

48 Suk, Ryan, Kaiping Liao, Cici X. Bauer, Catherine Basil, and Meng Li. "Human Papillomavirus Vaccine Administration Trends among Commercially Insured US Adults Aged 27-45 Years before and after Advisory Committee on Immunization Practices Recommendation Change, 2007-2020." *JAMA Health Forum* 3, no. 12 (December 16, 2022). https://doi.org/10.1001/jamahealthforum.2022.4716.

49 VRBPAC. "VRBPAC Background Document Gardasil™ HPV Quadrivalent Vaccine May 18, 2006 VRBPAC Meeting." Zenodo, May 18, 2006. https://doi.org/10.5281/zenodo.1434214.

50 Dunne, Eileen F., Elizabeth R. Unger, Maya Sternberg, Geraldine McQuillan, David C. Swan, Sonya S. Patel, and Lauri E. Markowitz. "Prevalence of HPV Infection among Females in the United States." *JAMA* 297, no. 8 (February 28, 2007): 813. https://doi.org/10.1001/jama.297.8.813.

51 Slade, Barbara A. "Postlicensure Safety Surveillance for Quadrivalent Human Papillomavirus Recombinant Vaccine." *JAMA* 302, no. 7 (August 19, 2009): 750. https://doi.org/10.1001/jama.2009.1201.

52 Ibid.

53 Ibid.

54 Tomljenovic, Lucija, Emily Tarsell, James Garrett, Christopher A. Shaw, and Mary S. Holland. "Significant Under-Reporting of Quadrivalent Human Papillomavirus Vaccine-Associated Serious Adverse Events in the United States: Time for Change? *Science, Public Health Policy, and The Law.* 2 (May 2021):37-58. https://cf5e727d-d029fe2d3ad957f.filesusr.com/ugd/adf864_2dede593f4a04e64ab6c0c45bc14d450.pdf.

55 Ibid.

56 U.S. Food and Drug Administration. "CFR—Code of Federal Regulations Title 21." October 17, 2023. https://www.accessdata.fda.gov/scripts/cdrh/cfdocs/cfcfr/cfrsearch.cfm?fr=312.32#.

57 "Cancer of the Cervix Uteri—Cancer Stat Facts." SEER. Accessed January 25, 2024. https://seer.cancer.gov/statfacts/html/cervix.html.

58 Ibid.

59 Issanov, Alpamys, Mohammad Karim, Gulzhanat Aimagambetova, and Trevor Dummer. "Does Vaccination Protect against Human Papillomavirus-Related Cancers? Preliminary Findings from the United States National Health and Nutrition Examination Survey (2011–2018)." *Vaccines* 10, no. 12 (December 10, 2022): 2113. https://doi.org/10.3390/vaccines10122113.

60 Ibid.

61 Hartman, Melissa. "Cervical Cancer Is Preventable." Johns Hopkins Bloomberg School of Public Health, January 24, 2023. https://publichealth.jhu.edu/2023/cervical-cancer-is-preventable.

62 https://jamanetwork.com/journals/jama/fullarticle/2697704.

63 Ibid.

64 Huang, Yu, Xinzhi Wu, Ying Lin, Wenzhou Li, Jiahua Liu, and Baozhi Song. "Multiple Sexual Partners and Vaginal Microecological Disorder Are Associated with HPV Infection and Cervical Carcinoma Development." *Oncology Letters* 20, no. 2 (June 16, 2020): 1915–21. https://doi.org/10.3892/ol.2020.11738.

65 "How Do Viruses Mutate and What it Means for a Vaccine?" Pfizer. 2024. https://www.pfizer.com/news/articles/how_do_viruses_mutate_and_what_it_means_for_a_vaccine.

66 Ibid.

67 Fischer, Sonja, Marcus Bettstetter, Andrea Becher, Marlene Lessel, Cyril Bank, Matthias Krams, Ingrid Becker, Arndt Haremann, Wolfgang Jagla, and Andreas Gaumann. "Shift in Prevalence of HPV Types in Cervical Cytology Specimens in the Era of HPV Vaccination." *Oncology Letters* 12, no. 1 (June 1, 2016): 601–10. https://doi.org/10.3892/ol.2016.4668.

68 Ibid.

69 Ibid.

70 Ibid.

71 Guo, Fangjian, Jacqueline M. Hirth, and Abbey B. Berenson. "Human Papillomavirus Vaccination and Pap Smear Uptake among Young Women in the United States: Role of Provider and Patient." *Journal of Women's Health* 26, no. 10 (October 2017): 1114–22. https://doi.org/10.1089/jwh.2017.6424.

Chapter 19

1 Notice of Voluntary Dismissal Pursuant To F.R.C.P. 41(A)(1)(A)(I). United States District Court Southern District Of New York. February 10, 2019. https://icandecide.org/wp-content/uploads/2019/09/ICAvFDA-Resolved-Court-Filed-Copy.pdf.

2 Mehrabadi, Azar, Linda Dodds, Noni E. MacDonald, Karina A. Top, Eric I. Benchimol, Jeffrey C. Kwong, Justin R. Ortiz, et al. "Association of Maternal Influenza Vaccination during Pregnancy with Early Childhood Health Outcomes." *JAMA* 325, no. 22 (June 8, 2021): 2285. https://doi.org/10.1001/jama.2021.6778.

3 Donahue, James G., Burney A. Kieke, Jennifer P. King, Frank DeStefano, Maria A. Mascola, Stephanie A. Irving, T. Craig Cheetham, et al. "Association of Spontaneous Abortion with Receipt of Inactivated Influenza Vaccine Containing H1n1pdm09 in 2010–11 and 2011–12." *Vaccine* 35, no. 40 (September 2017): 5314–22. https://doi.org/10.1016/j.vaccine.2017.06.069.

4 Pahwa, Roma, Amandeep Goyal, and Ishwarlal Jialal. "Chronic Inflammation." Section. In StatPearls [Internet]. Treasure Island, FL: StatPearls Publishing, 2023. https://www.ncbi.nlm.nih.gov/books/NBK493173/.

5 Christian, Lisa M., Jay D. Iams, Kyle Porter, and Ronald Glaser. "Inflammatory Responses to Trivalent Influenza Virus Vaccine among Pregnant Women." *Vaccine* 29, no. 48 (November 2011): 8982–87. https://doi.org/10.1016/j.vaccine.2011.09.039.

6 Brown, A. S., A. Sourander, S. Hinkka-Yli-Salomäki, I. W. McKeague, J. Sundvall, and H.M. Surcel. "Elevated Maternal C-Reactive Protein and Autism in a National

Birth Cohort." *Molecular Psychiatry* 19, no. 2 (January 22, 2013): 259–64. https://doi.org/10.1038/mp.2012.197.

7 Zawadzka, Aleksandra, Magdalena Cieślik, and Agata Adamczyk. "The Role of Maternal Immune Activation in the Pathogenesis of Autism: A Review of the Evidence, Proposed Mechanisms and Implications for Treatment." *International Journal of Molecular Sciences* 22, no. 21 (October 26, 2021): 11516. https://doi.org/10.3390/ijms222111516.

8 Trotta, F., R. Da Cas, S. Spila Alegiani, M. Gramegna, M. Venegoni, C. Zocchetti, and G. Traversa. "Evaluation of Safety Of A/H1N1 Pandemic Vaccination during Pregnancy: Cohort Study." *BMJ* 348, no. May29 5 (May 29, 2014). https://doi.org/10.1136/bmj.g3361.

9 Chung, Jessie R., Sara S. Kim, Rebecca J. Kondor, Catherine Smith, Alicia P. Budd, Sara Y. Tartof, Ana Florea, et al. "Interim Estimates of 2021–22 Seasonal Influenza Vaccine Effectiveness — United States, February 2022." *Morbidity and Mortality Weekly Report* 71, no. 10 (March 11, 2022): 365–70. https://doi.org/10.15585/mmwr.mm7110a1.

10 Tenforde, Mark W., Zachary A. Weber, Duck-Hye Yang, Malini B. DeSilva, Kristin Dascomb, Stephanie A. Irving, Allison L. Naleway, et al. "Influenza Vaccine Effectiveness against Influenza A–Associated Emergency Department, Urgent Care, and Hospitalization Encounters among Us Adults, 2022–2023." *Journal of Infectious Diseases*, December 2, 2023. https://doi.org/10.1093/infdis/jiad542.

11 Bi, Qifang, Barbra A. Dickerman, Huong Q. McLean, Emily T. Martin, Manjusha Gaglani, Karen J. Wernli, G.K. Balasubramani, Brendan Flannery, Marc Lipsitch, and Sarah Cobey. "Reduced effectiveness of repeat influenza vaccination: Distinguishing among within-season waning, recent clinical infection, and subclinical infection." *MedRxiv,* Preprint. September 27th, 2023. MedRiv. https://doi.org/10.1101/2023.03.12.23287173.

12 Ibid.

13 Murray, Terry. "Repeated flu shots may blunt effectiveness." *CMAJ*. 187 no. 6. (April 7, 2015). https://www.cmaj.ca/content/187/6/E180.

14 Ibid.

15 Khurana, Surender, Megan Hahn, Elizabeth M. Coyle, Lisa R. King, Tsai-Lien Lin, John Treanor, Andrea Sant, and Hana Golding. "Repeat Vaccination Reduces Antibody Affinity Maturation across Different Influenza Vaccine Platforms in Humans." *Nature Communications* 10, no. 1 (July 26, 2019). https://doi.org/10.1038/s41467-019-11296-5.

16 "Influenza Vaccine Market Size: Growth Analysis Report [2030]." Market Research Report. July 2023. https://www.fortunebusinessinsights.com/industry-reports/influenza-vaccine-market-101896.

17 Fowlkes, Ashley L., Francisco Nogareda, Annette Regan, Sergio Loayza, Jose Mendez Mancio, Lindsey M. Duca, Paula Couto, et al. "Interim Effectiveness Estimates of 2023 Southern Hemisphere Influenza Vaccines in Preventing Influenza-Associated Hospitalizations — REVELAC–I Network, March–July

2023." *Morbidity and Mortality Weekly Report* 72, no. 37 (September 15, 2023): 1010–15. https://doi.org/10.15585/mmwr.mm7237e1.

18 "Vaccine Safety for Moms-to-Be." Centers for Disease Control and Prevention, November 22, 2021. https://www.cdc.gov/vaccines/pregnancy/vacc-safety.html.

19 Thorp, Maggie, and Jim Thorp. "FOIA Reveals Troubling Relationship between HHS/CDC & ACOG." America Out Loud News, May 27, 2023. https://www.americaoutloud.news/foia-reveals-troubling-relationship-between-hhs-cdc-the-american-college-of-obstetricians-and-gynecologists/.

20 "Covid-19 Community Corps." COVID.gov, February 16, 2023. https://www.covid.gov/get-involved/community-corps.

21 "Pregnant and Protected from Covid-19." CDC Foundation. Accessed January 26, 2024. https://www.cdcfoundation.org/pregnant-and-protected.

22 Goh, Orlanda, Deanette Pang, Janice Tan, David Lye, Chia Yin Chong, Benjamin Ong, Kelvin Bryan Tan, and Chee Fu Yung. "MRNA SARS-COV-2 Vaccination before vs during Pregnancy and Omicron Infection among Infants." *JAMA Network Open* 6, no. 11 (November 10, 2023). https://doi.org/10.1001/jamanetworkopen.2023.42475.

23 Greene, Jenna. "'Paramount Importance': Judge Orders FDA to Hasten Release . . ." Reuters, January 7, 2022. https://www.reuters.com/legal/government/paramount-importance-judge-orders-fda-hasten-release-pfizer-vaccine-docs-2022-01-07/.

24 Kelly, Amy. "Report 69: Bombshell—Pfizer and FDA Knew in Early 2021 That Pfizer Mrna COVID 'Vaccine' Caused Dire Fetal and Infant Risks, Including Death. They Began an Aggressive Campaign to Vaccinate Pregnant Women Anyway." DailyClout, April 29, 2023. https://dailyclout.io/bombshell-pfizer-and-the-fda-knew-in-early-2021-that-the-pfizer-mrna-covid-vaccine-caused-dire-fetal-and-infant-risks-they-began-an-aggressive-campaign-to-vaccinate-pregnant-women-anyway/.

25 "Pregnancy and Lactation Cumulative Review." Public Health and Medical Professionals for Transparency. April 20, 2021. https://www.phmpt.org/wp-content/uploads/2023/04/125742_S2_M1_pllr-cumulative-review.pdf.

26 Van Spall, Harriette Gillian. "Exclusion of Pregnant and Lactating Women from Covid-19 Vaccine Trials: A Missed Opportunity." *European Heart Journal*, March 4, 2021. https://doi.org/10.1093/eurheartj/ehab103.

27 "04/23/21: Press Briefing by White House COVID-19 Response Team and Public Health Officials." YouTube, April 23, 2021. https://www.youtube.com/watch?v=kbdoXen3AR8.

28 Shimabukuro, Tom T., Shin Y. Kim, Tanya R. Myers, Pedro L. Moro, Titilope Oduyebo, Lakshmi Panagiotakopoulos, Paige L. Marquez, et al. "Preliminary Findings of Mrna COVID-19 Vaccine Safety in Pregnant Persons." *New England Journal of Medicine* 384, no. 24 (June 17, 2021): 2273–82. https://doi.org/10.1056/nejmoa2104983.

29 Sun, Hong. "On Preliminary Findings of Mrna COVID-19 Vaccine Safety in Pregnant Persons." Correspondence. *New England Journal of Medicine* 385, no. 16 (October 14, 2021): 1535–36. https://doi.org/10.1056/nejmc2113516.

30 Velez, Maria P., Deshayne B. Fell, Jonas P. Shellenberger, Jeffrey C. Kwong, and Joel G. Ray. "Miscarriage after SARS-COV-2 Vaccination: A Population-based Cohort Study." *BJOG: An International Journal of Obstetrics & Gynaecology*, November 16, 2023. https://doi.org/10.1111/1471-0528.17721.

31 Lin, Xinhua, Bishoy Botros, Monica Hanna, Ellen Gurzenda, Claudia Manzano De Mejia, Martin Chavez, and Nazeeh Hanna. "Transplacental Transmission of the COVID-19 Vaccine Mrna: Evidence from Placental, Maternal and Cord Blood Analyses Post-Vaccination." A*merican Journal of Obstetrics and Gynecology,* 2024.

32 "Assessment Report COVID-19 Vaccine Moderna." European Medicines Agency. March 11, 2021. https://www.ema.europa.eu/en/documents/assessment-report/spikevax-previously-covid-19-vaccine-moderna-epar-public-assessment-report_en.pdf.

33 Lin, Xinhua, Bishoy Botros, Monica Hanna, Ellen Gurzenda, Claudia Manzano De Mejia, Martin Chavez, and Nazeeh Hanna. "Transplacental Transmission of the COVID-19 Vaccine Mrna: Evidence from Placental, Maternal and Cord Blood Analyses Post-Vaccination." A*merican Journal of Obstetrics and Gynecology,* 2024.

34 Chudov, Igor. "How to Make Covid Vaccines Appear to Be 'Safe for Pregnancy.'" How to Make COVID Vaccines Appear to be "Safe for Pregnancy," November 15, 2023. https://www.igor-chudov.com/p/how-to-make-covid-vaccines-appear?utm_source=profile&utm_medium=reader2.

35 Ibid.

36 Rahmati, Masoud, Dong Keon Yon, Seung Won Lee, Laurie Butler, Ai Koyanagi, Louis Jacob, Jae Il Shin, and Lee Smith. "Effects of Covid-19 Vaccination during Pregnancy on SARS-COV-2 Infection and Maternal and Neonatal Outcomes: A Systematic Review and Meta-analysis." *Reviews in Medical Virology* 33, no. 3 (March 10, 2023). https://doi.org/10.1002/rmv.2434.

37 Buergin, Natacha, Pedro Lopez-Ayala, Julia R. Hirsiger, Philip Mueller, Daniela Median, Noemi Glarner, Klara Rumora, et al. "Sex-specific Differences in Myocardial Injury Incidence after Covid-19 Mrna-1273 Booster Vaccination." *European Journal of Heart Failure* 25, no. 10 (August 9, 2023): 1871–81. https://doi.org/10.1002/ejhf.2978.

38 Hall, Michael E., Eric M. George, and Joey P. Granger. "El Corazón Durante El Embarazo." *Revista Española de Cardiología* 64, no. 11 (November 2011): 1045–50. https://doi.org/10.1016/j.recesp.2011.07.009.

39 Ibid.

40 Martinez, Sara C., and Sharonne N. Hayes. "Ischemic Complications of Pregnancy: Who Is at Risk?" *US Cardiology Review* 10, no. 1 (2016): 14. https://doi.org/10.15420/usc.2016.10.1.14.

41 Kotit, Susy, and Magdi Yacoub. "Cardiovascular Adverse Events in Pregnancy: A Global Perspective." *Global Cardiology Science and Practice* 2021, no. 1 (April 30, 2021). https://doi.org/10.21542/gcsp.2021.5.

42 Sanofi Pasteur Limited. *Package Insert: ADACEL*. Food and Drug Administration (FDA), 2023. https://www.fda.gov/media/119862/download.

43 GlaxoSmithKline Biologicals. Package Insert: BOOSTRIX. Food and Drug Administration (FDA), 2023. https://www.fda.gov/media/124002/download.

44 Lee, Lucia. Clinical Review Memo: BOOSTRIX. https://www.fda.gov/media/162830/download.

45 GlaxoSmithKline Biologicals. Package Insert: BOOSTRIX. Food and Drug Administration (FDA), 2023. https://www.fda.gov/media/124002/download.

46 Hardy-Fairbanks, Abbey J., Stephanie J. Pan, Michael D. Decker, David R. Johnson, David P. Greenberg, Kathryn B. Kirkland, Elizabeth A. Talbot, and Henry H. Bernstein. "Immune Responses in Infants Whose Mothers Received Tdap Vaccine during Pregnancy." *Pediatric Infectious Disease Journal* 32, no. 11 (November 2013): 1257–60. https://doi.org/10.1097/inf.0b013e3182a09b6a.

47 Florea, Ana, Lina S. Sy, Bradley K. Ackerson, Lei Qian, Yi Luo, Tracy Becerra-Culqui, Gina S. Lee, et al. "Investigating Tetanus, Diphtheria, Acellular Pertussis Vaccination during Pregnancy and Risk of Congenital Anomalies." *Infectious Diseases and Therapy* 12, no. 2 (December 15, 2022): 411–23. https://doi.org/10.1007/s40121-022-00731-8.

48 Lee, Lucia. Clinical Review Memo: BOOSTRIX. https://www.fda.gov/media/162830/download.

49 GlaxoSmithKline Biologicals. Package Insert: BOOSTRIX. Food and Drug Administration (FDA), 2023. https://www.fda.gov/media/124002/download.

50 "Use of the Pfizer Respiratory Syncytial Virus Vaccine during Pregnancy for the Prevention of Respiratory Syncytial Virus–Associated Lower Respiratory Tract Disease in Infants: Recommendations of the Advisory Committee on Immunization Practices—United States, 2023." Centers for Disease Control and Prevention, October 6, 2023. https://www.cdc.gov/mmwr/volumes/72/wr/mm7241e1.htm.

51 Office of the Commissioner. "FDA Approves First Vaccine for Pregnant Individuals to Prevent RSV in Infants." U.S. Food and Drug Administration. August 21, 2023. Accessed January 26, 2024. https://www.fda.gov/news-events/press-announcements/fda-approves-first-vaccine-pregnant-individuals-prevent-rsv-infants.

52 "RSV (Respiratory Syncytial Virus)." Centers for Disease Control and Prevention, November 7, 2023. https://www.cdc.gov/rsv/index.html.

53 Li, You, Xin Wang, Dianna M. Blau, Mauricio T. Caballero, Daniel R. Feikin, Christopher J. Gill, Shabir A. Madhi, et al. "Global, Regional, and National Disease Burden Estimates of Acute Lower Respiratory Infections Due to Respiratory Syncytial Virus in Children Younger than 5 Years in 2019: A Systematic Analysis." *The Lancet* 399, no. 10340 (May 2022): 2047–64. https://doi.org/10.1016/s0140-6736(22)00478-0.

54 Hamid, Sarah, Amber Winn, Rishika Parikh, Jefferson M. Jones, Meredith McMorrow, Mila M. Prill, Benjamin J. Silk, Heather M. Scobie, and Aron J. Hall. "Seasonality of Respiratory Syncytial Virus — United States, 2017–2023." *Morbidity and Mortality Weekly Report* 72, no. 14 (April 7, 2023): 355–61. https://doi.org/10.15585/mmwr.mm7214a1.

55 “GSK Provides Further Update on Phase III RSV Maternal Vaccine Candidate Programme.” GlaxoSmithKline, February 28, 2022. https://www.gsk.com/en-gb/media/press-releases/gsk-provides-further-update-on-phase-iii-rsv-maternal-vaccine-candidate-programme/.

56 “Vaccines and Related Biological Products Advisory Committee.” Sponsor Briefing Document; Meeting. GlaxoSmithKline. February 28—March 1 2023. https://www.fda.gov/media/165621/download#page=42.

57 Boytchev, Hristio. “Concerns over Informed Consent for Pregnant Women in Pfizer’s RSV Vaccine Trial.” *BMJ*, November 15, 2023. https://doi.org/10.1136/bmj.p2620.

58 “The BMJ investigates concerns over informed consent for pregnant women in Pfizer’s RSV vaccine trial.” BMJ Publishing Group Ltd. NOvember 16, 2023. https://www.bmj.com/company/newsroom/the-bmj-investigates-concerns-over-informed-consent-for-pregnant-women-in-pfizers-rsv-vaccine-trial/.

59 Fleming-Dutra, Katherine E., Jefferson M. Jones, Lauren E. Roper, Mila M. Prill, Ismael R. Ortega-Sanchez, Danielle L. Moulia, Megan Wallace, et al. “Use of the Pfizer Respiratory Syncytial Virus Vaccine during Pregnancy for the Prevention of Respiratory Syncytial Virus–Associated Lower Respiratory Tract Disease in Infants: Recommendations of the Advisory Committee on Immunization Practices — United States, 2023.” *Morbidity and Mortality Weekly Report* 72, no. 41 (October 13, 2023): 1115–22. https://doi.org/10.15585/mmwr.mm7241e1.

60 “Preterm Birth.” World Health Organization. Accessed January 26, 2024. https://www.who.int/news-room/fact-sheets/detail/preterm-birth.

61 Manuck, Tracy A., Madeline Murguia Rice, Jennifer L. Bailit, William A. Grobman, Uma M. Reddy, Ronald J. Wapner, John M. Thorp, et al. “Preterm Neonatal Morbidity and Mortality by Gestational Age: A Contemporary Cohort.” *American Journal of Obstetrics and Gynecology* 215, no. 1 (July 2016). https://doi.org/10.1016/j.ajog.2016.01.004.

62 K. C., Anil, Prem Lal Basel, and Sarswoti Singh. “Low Birth Weight and Its Associated Risk Factors: Health Facility-Based Case-Control Study.” *PLOS ONE* 15, no. 6 (June 22, 2020). https://doi.org/10.1371/journal.pone.0234907.

63 “What Are Jaundice and Kernicterus?” Centers for Disease Control and Prevention, CDC Archives. December 8, 2020. https://archive.cdc.gov/#/details?url=https://www.cdc.gov/ncbddd/jaundice/facts.html.

64 “What Are the Risks of Preeclampsia & Eclampsia to the Mother?” Eunice Kennedy Shriver National Institute of Child Health and Human Development, November 19, 2018. https://www.nichd.nih.gov/health/topics/preeclampsia/conditioninfo/risk-mother.

65 Dimitriadis, Evdokia, Daniel L. Rolnik, Wei Zhou, Guadalupe Estrada-Gutierrez, Kaori Koga, Rossana P. Francisco, Clare Whitehead, et al. “Pre-Eclampsia.” *Nature Reviews Disease Primers* 9, no. 1 (February 16, 2023). https://doi.org/10.1038/s41572-023-00417-6.

66 Pittara, T., A. Vyrides, D. Lamnisos, and K. Giannakou. “Pre-eclampsia and Long-term Health Outcomes for Mother and Infant: An Umbrella Review.” *BJOG: An*

International Journal of Obstetrics & Gynaecology 128, no. 9 (March 23, 2021): 1421–30. https://doi.org/10.1111/1471-0528.16683.

67 Ibid.

68 Sonja A. Rasmussen, Denise J. Jamieson. "Maternal RSV Vaccine—Weighing Risks and Benefits." New England Journal of Medicine, 390, 11, 91050-1052). March 13, 2024.

69 Pittara, T., A. Vyrides, D. Lamnisos, and K. Giannakou. "Pre-eclampsia and Long-term Health Outcomes for Mother and Infant: An Umbrella Review." *BJOG: An International Journal of Obstetrics & Gynaecology* 128, no. 9 (March 23, 2021): 1421–30. https://doi.org/10.1111/1471-0528.16683.

Chapter 20

1 Sayki, Inci. "Despite Record Federal Lobbying Spending, the Pharmaceutical and Health Product Industry Lost Their Biggest Legislative Bet in 2022." OpenSecrets News, February 2, 2023. https://www.opensecrets.org/news/2023/02/despite-record-federal-lobbying-spending-the-pharmaceutical-and-health-product-industry-lost-their-biggest-legislative-bet-in-2022.

2 "VFC: Vaccines for Children Program." Centers for Disease Control and Prevention, October 24, 2022. https://www.cdc.gov/vaccines/programs/vfc/index.html.

Chapter 21

1 Thornton, Russell G. "The Learned Intermediary Doctrine and Its Effects on Prescribing Physicians." *Baylor University Medical Center Proceedings* 16, no. 3 (July 2003): 359–61. https://doi.org/10.1080/08998280.2003.11927929.

2 National Research Council (US) Division of Health Promotion and Disease Prevention. "Liability for the Production and Sale of Vaccines." Chapter. In Vaccine Supply and Innovation. Washington, DC: National Academies Press (US), 1985.

3 "History of Vaccine Information Statements." U.S. Department of Health and Human Services. Centers for Disease Control and Prevention. Accessed January 20, 2024. https://www.cdc.gov/vaccines/hcp/vis/downloads/vis-history.pdf.

4 Ibid.

5 "Covid-19 Vaccine EUA Recipient/Caregiver Fact Sheets." Centers for Disease Control and Prevention, September 28, 2023.

6 The Belmont Report: Ethical principles and guidelines for the Protection of Human Subjects of Research. 1978. US Department of Health and Human Services. https://www.hhs.gov/ohrp/regulations-and-policy/belmont-report/read-the-belmont-report/index.html.

7 Ibid.

8 COVID-19 Vaccine Consent Form. Centers for Disease Control and Prevention. September 22, 2021. https://www.cdc.gov/flu/school/slv/support.htm.

9 COVID-19 Vaccine Consent Form. Walgreens. February 03, 2021. https://www.walgreens.com/images/adaptive/si/pdf/1624373-0331_FY21_COVID19_VAR_OffSite_ENG.pdf.

10 674 COVID-19 Vaccine Consent Form. ca.gov. Accessed January 20, 2024. https://www.cdph.ca.gov/Programs/CID/DCDC/CDPH%20Document%20Library/COVID-19/Pfizer-Minor-Consent-Form-Sample-INT-PDF-ADA.pdf.

11 Coulter, Harris, and Barbara Fisher. 1991. *In A Shot in the Dark*, 83. New York, NY: Avery.

12 Vivek H. Murthy, Surgeon General, et al. vs Missouri, et al., "Brief Of American Academy Of Pediatrics, American Medical Association, American Academy Of Family Physicians, American College Of Physicians, And American Geriatrics Society As Amici Curiae in Support Of Petitioners." Accessed January 20, 2024. https://www.supremecourt.gov/DocketPDF/23/23-411/294091/20231222102540387_FINAL%20Murthy%20Amicus%20for%20filing.pdf?utm_source=substack&utm_medium=email.

13 Ibid.

14 Diekema, Douglas S. "Responding to Parental Refusals of Immunization of Children." *Pediatrics* 115, no. 5 (May 1, 2005): 1428–31. https://doi.org/10.1542/peds.2005-0316.

15 Edwards, Kathryn M., and Jesse M. Hackell. "Countering Vaccine Hesitancy." *Pediatrics* 138, no. 3 (September 1, 2016).

16 Garcia, Tamara B., and Sean T. O'Leary. "Dismissal Policies for Vaccine Refusal among US Physicians: A Literature Review." *Human Vaccines & Immunotherapeutics* 16, no. 5 (February 20, 2020): 1189–93.

Chapter 22

1 Fenner, F. "Global Eradication of Smallpox." *Clinical Infectious Diseases* 4, no. 5 (September 1, 1982): 916–30. https://doi.org/10.1093/clinids/4.5.916.

2 Morabito, Charlotte. "How HIV Research Paved the Way for the Covid Mrna Vaccines." CNBC, December 1, 2021. https://www.cnbc.com/2021/12/01/how-hiv-research-paved-the-way-for-the-covid-mrna-vaccines.html?&qsearchterm=HIV+r.

3 Institute of Medicine. *The Childhood Immunization Schedule and Safety: Stakeholder Concerns, Scientific Evidence, and Future Studies.* Washington, DC: The National Academies Press. 2013. https://doi.org/10.17226/13563.

Index

S

T

V

Z

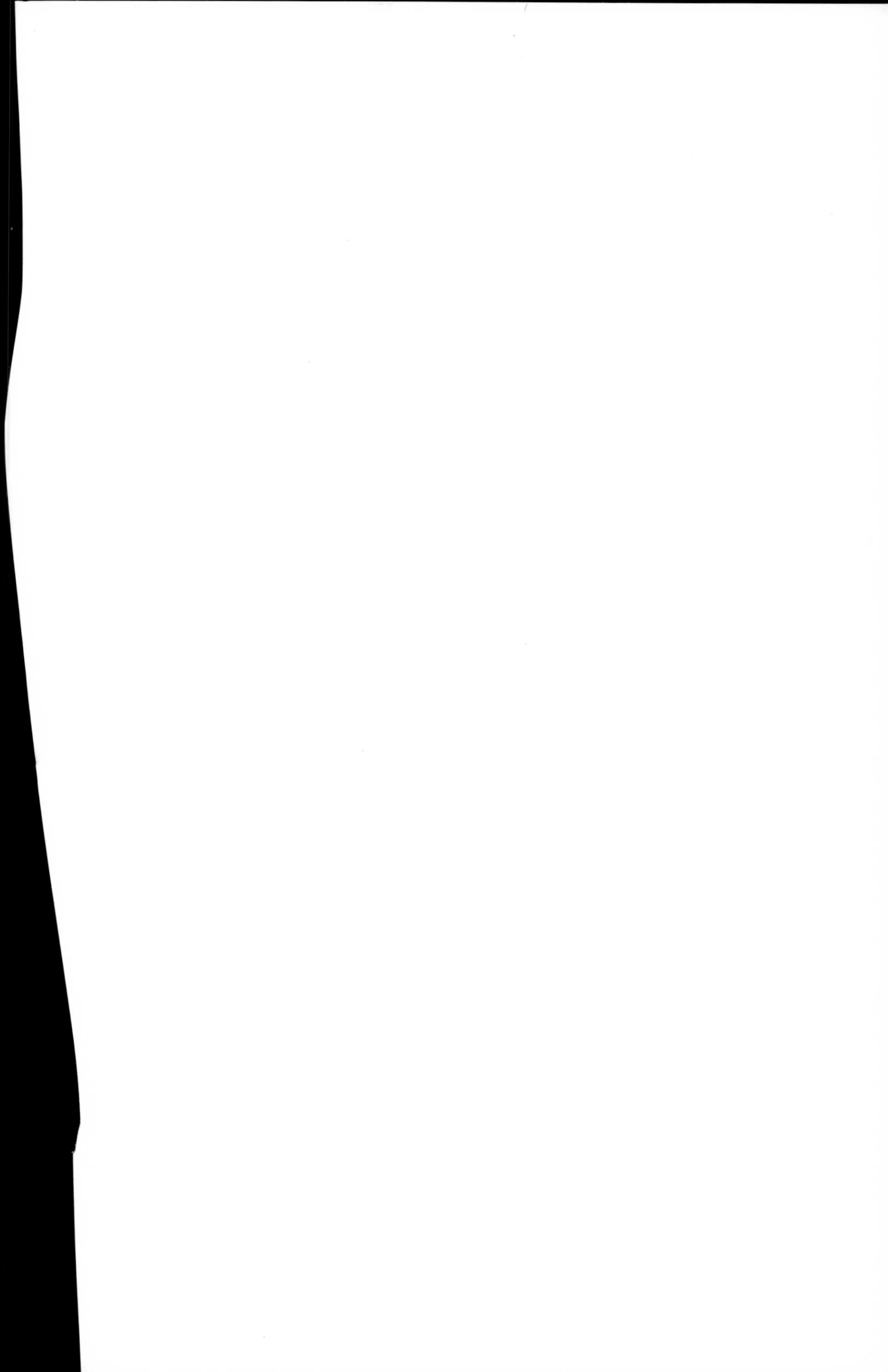